Fatal

Advice

Edited by Michèle Aina Barale, Jonathan Goldberg,

Michael Moon, and Eve Kosofsky Sedgwick

Fatal Advice

Advice

HOW SAFE-SEX EDUCATION WENT WRONG

Cindy Patton

Duke University Press Durham and London

1996

© 1996 Duke University Press

All rights reserved

Printed in the United States of America on acid-free paper ∞

Typeset in Times Roman with Modern Torino display

by Keystone Typesetting, Inc.

Library of Congress Cataloging-in-Publication Data

appear on the last printed page

of this book.

Want to know a dirty little secret?
Condoms don't save lives.

But restraint does.
Only fools think condoms are foolproof.
Remember, better safe than sorry.

Some common sense and a public service announcement
from the Catholic League for Religious and Civil Rights
1011 First Avenue, New York, NY 10022
(212) 371-3191

---

*Advertisement in the New York City subways appearing in
June 1994, during the celebration of the 25th anniversary of
the Stonewall riots, which sparked the contemporary
gay liberation movement.*

Contents

Acknowledgments

This volume contains work produced over the past seven years, including sections of previously published works that have been substantially revised and reframed, and augmented by new work that makes a larger argument than was possible in any earlier essay. Reworking the material has been a protracted and emotional task. I have had the opportunity to see how much my own thinking has changed as events and projects have come and gone, but these changes also remind me that some of the people who were important to me and to this work will not get to see the finished project. I want to make a special dedication to three of those people here: to Michael Lynch, a crucial member of Toronto's *The Body Politics* collective, gay historian, archivist, and poet; to Al Parker, whose career and strong advocacy of safe sex within the porn industry made possible some of the texts I discuss in chapter 3 — I especially recall his generous help in launching Safe Company for the gay men of Boston; to Mike Reagle, who introduced me to both poststructuralism and the bushes, who struggled for the rights of prisoners, and especially their right to information about HIV, means of preventing transmission, and access to care.

I want to also thank Judy Frank, who, for the entire course of these writings, got me up many hills and through several swampy valleys; Eve Kosofsky Sedgwick, who continues to be at the center of my pretended-extended family; Mary Petty, who convinced me that work isn't everything, that love matters, and tolerated my laptop companion on numerous vacations; Carlos Cano, who was a mainstay of emotional support, a running partner, and confidant of the early 1990s; Lisa Duggan, for helping to tackle various flying monsters — bats out of hell and illusory magpies; and my little dog Alex, who always wants to be happy, and who provides an invaluable alternate perspective on life. Sadly, this book will not appear in a canine translation.

The following people had significant involvement in earlier phases of the work that I have rewritten for this volume: Douglas Crimp, Diana Fuss, Larry Gross, Lisa Henderson, Ken Morrison, Don Moss, Jenny Terry, Jackie Urla, Carole Vance, and Tom Waugh. I especially thank Jonathan Goldberg, Michael Moon, Eve Kosofsky Sedgwick, Michèle Barale, and Ken Wissoker for their enthusiasm for the project, despite the many delays that resulted from my decision to join the academy, with concomitant distractions, and Katie Kent for her keen eye and willingness to conquer my grammatical oddities.

The Humanities Research Center at the Australian National University in Canberra, Australia, and especially John Ballard and Jill Matthews, provided me with the time and incredibly beautiful environment in which to work on this manuscript.

1

Around 1989

In 1989, an attentive gay male student helped me cue the video for a paper I was about to give on heterosexual pornography.[1] As a closeup shot ended, and the camera panned back to lovingly capture the come shot, the young man shrieked in distress.

"It's a man and a *woman!*" he exclaimed. "And they're practicing safe sex!"

I began to explain that "pulling out" was necessary to the "come shot,"[2] the cinematic mark of male orgasm that has been conventional in pornography since the 1970s. Predating the very idea of safe sex by more than a decade, the come shot was meant to signify the truth of male orgasm, not the distance of the event from "coming inside."[3] For me, the idea of fucking without a condom was antithetical to the safe sex messages I had worked for some years to perfect. For my young friend, the practice he observed met the minimal requirement of at least one safe sex dictum: on me, not in me. For him, two men performing the come shot were not only practicing safe sex, they were demonstrating it: what ostensibly gay men did in films was not only real, but didactic. His only surprise was that heterosexuals had somehow copied gay men, now America's safe sex trendsetters.

Not long after this experience I had a second collision with variant intracommunity interpretations, this time writ large as a controversy over a sexually explicit safe sex advertisement that had been placed in *GO*, the gay and lesbian community newspaper of Ottawa.[4] The ad (which was, in my view, tasteful in the extreme) featured a frontally nude male sporting a condom on his not very hard cock. The ad had been produced by a local gay male photographer in conjunction with Ottawa's AIDS education council. The photographer's work — portraiture, erotica, news photography, and, by 1989, safe sex posters — was widely recognizable in the local community: a Phillip Hannan photograph was as natural in queer Ottawa as a Keith Haring drawing in New York City.

But this particular photograph created controversy on two fronts: in order to make the ad more acceptable in the pages of a community newspaper — in order to make the ad visually distinct from, say, pornography or bar ads — Hannan had agreed to photograph the model at half mast. Radical feminists were outraged by the appearance of even a didactic dick in the pages of their local rag, and safe sex pedagogues were concerned that the dick wasn't hard *enough*. They feared that novices might try to apply a condom before a proper erection. Poor Phillip was caught in the middle.

The group of lesbians who levied the strongest accusations deemed the ad pornographic, invoking the wealth of controversial analysis about the role of such representations in the oppression of women. As a depiction of male sexuality, they argued, the ad was assaultive to women, especially to female victims of male sexual violence. Although this hard-line antiporn position was only a small voice in the larger lesbian and gay community, other women felt torn by a more inarticulate discomfort with the ad. Some wanted to maintain their allegiance to their sisters, and yet other women simply weren't interested in having naked men in their community newspaper. The women who had approved the ad had initially believed that it constituted valid risk reduction education. Now they wondered if they had gone too far.

The controversy centered on variant theories of representation and their political implications for promoting safe sex. In a conversation with one of the women who took the radical feminist position, I discovered how the conviction that pornography causes negative behaviors aligned with the view that multiple partnering is a slippery slope to high-risk sex. The woman emphasized that objecting to the ad did not mean that she opposed risk reduction education. Quite the contrary, she equated monogamy with safe sex and believed men should work toward "deeper," "committed" relationships.

Far from eroticizing safe sex, she argued, viewing pornography (including Hannan's safe sex photos) leads to uncaring, promiscuous relationships.

"What exactly did you feel was wrong about this ad," I asked.

"It had exposed male genitals," she said.

"Oh," I said, with an air of confusion. "I thought you said he was *wearing* a condom."

On one hand, I understood these women's interpretation of the penis as a potential weapon: a brandished penis signified the danger of misogynist violence. But after years of working on safe sex projects, I now understood that danger lurked in the body fluid that the erect penis foretold: a penis dressed in a condom was a penis made safe.

I do not retell these stories in order to suggest that gay men's lives are more at risk than the lives of the women whom the radical feminists were concerned to protect.[5] Nor do I mean to sentimentalize my young friend's complicated misrecognition. But these incidents, in different ways, brought home the stakes in and complexities of representations of sexuality. As both stories suggest, a range of groups, for nearly opposite reasons, have placed great stock in pornography's power to direct human behavior. One branch of feminists concerned about violence against women hoped to link pornography watching with the propensity to commit sexual violence. Equivalently, HIV prevention workers hoped that gay men would shift their desires and practices toward non–HIV-transmitting activities after imitating the "good" parts of safe sex pornography. But if the vast majority of heterosexual men who use pornography have never engaged in acts of sexual violence, then neither does safe sex pornography seem to impel audiences to commit acts of transmission disruption. Heterosexual men have not embarked on mass rampages of sexual violence after viewing the typical pornographic offerings, nor have anguished gay men found their sexual future in the lifesaving, utopian safe sex pornography. And yet, accusations based in the supposed power of pornography abound, despite the difficulty in claiming direct harms or benefits from viewing pornography.

There may well be a complex relationship between the genre of pornography and the systematic, largely negative representation of women in mass culture, just as there may well be imitative responses to countercultural or

Around 1989

5

interventionist sexual representations. But, personal testimonials notwith-standing, it seems unlikely that people widely imitate pornography in any straightforward way. If that were true, analysts would have to explain why some, but not all, pornographic images are imitated: in the de rigueur come shot of pornography, the insertive male pulls out of his partner to spew his semen. In "real life," few heterosexual men imitate this most basic and consistent feature of pornography. And, tragically, neither do many gay men. Moreover, condoms appear to have made only modest gains despite their visibility in mainstream gay porn and their status as the most common sym-bol of safe sex educational campaigns aimed at gay men. It is hard to make good on the strong claims that pornography is the hope for safe sex education or the cornerstone of misogyny. Pornographic safe sex projects may be worth pursuing, but not for the reasons usually proposed. In the last chapter I will suggest some of the ways radical safe sex projects might navigate the com-plex and variable interpretation of sexual representation in ways that shift the focus of discussion away from producing safe sex advice and toward inter-rogating the means of experiencing and reworking sexuality.

This book is particularly concerned to link varying ideas about safe sex through the early 1990s, especially as these imagined a sharp division be-tween those who were continuing to become infected and those who believed they could never be infected. A word or two about some of the concepts will be useful here: the idea of a national public is meant to indicate the collective who are represented as the proper citizens of a nation — here, the United States — an image that people may strive for or reject, but that is, evolving though it may be, the representational site of a struggle or negotiation over who it is that a government is supposed to govern. The citizen is the individ-ual case of the proper subject of the government, especially insofar as the citizen is the individual who responds to being governed without much fuss or clear policing. Safe sex is a term that I will constantly problematize. Although I will indicate from time to time the kinds of epidemiologic information that I believe accurately reflects the process of HIV transmission, I will use safe sex descriptively to refer to whatever different campaigns were promoting under the term. I want to make clear how variable were the meanings of "safe sex," not just as epidemiologists disagreed on their transmission data, but more important, as the various strategies for policing, reshaping, and politicizing sexuality converged under this initially innocent enough term. Finally, I distinguish between a national pedagogy, education, and organizing. The first is the mechanisms and logics that frame the evolving concept of citizen. Education refers to practices that make relatively sharp distinctions between those who know and teach and those who do not know and learn. Organizing refers to practices aimed at shaping and directing communities or subcultures in an effort to increase collective and individual viability.

Red Ribbons versus Safe Sex

As my opening stories suggest, by 1989 there were competing interpretations of what constituted safe sex and of who was supposed to practice it. But the multiple meanings available in pamphlets, films, even in the words "safe sex" (as opposed to . . . ?) and their interpretation by specific subcommunities were not merely intellectual fodder for the growing little industry of AIDS cultural critics. This play of meanings had dire consequences for those people who did not think that this advice applied to *them,* who deduced that they need not engage in transmission-interrupting techniques. Confusion about safe sex was bound up with the instability of sexual meanings more generally. "Safe sex" held symbolic utility for a country salvaging its failing identity in the face of a transnational, capitalist, global village culture that threatened (and still threatens) to make the very idea of a nation obsolete. If post-1960s America was in crisis already, the AIDS epidemic became a vehicle through which to renegotiate the meaning of being a good American.

The meaning of citizenship, who are to be counted as the true bearers of America's destiny and promise, undergoes revision as society and the state fail to make good on the complex, and also evolving, fantasy of what America *is.* The crisis surrounding the HIV epidemic exposed America's racism and homophobia in new ways, laying bare the ugly truth that the structure of benevolence — social programs, especially health care — simply were not meant for everyone. America needed a new model for the citizen, a tough love citizen who could be resolute about cutting federal funding without seeming cruel toward the burgeoning and increasingly organized group of people concerned about HIV whose only hope for treatment and care lay with a coordinated, well-funded federal response. By 1990, this new citizen of the national public had congealed as the opposite of the dangerous deviants who had become visible as "communities." At first, the new idea of citizen seemed only to apply to issues surrounding AIDS. However, as debates about health care and social welfare reform heated up in the 1992 presidential campaign, it became clear that the once liberal, now tough love citizen would be the inheritor of a mantle of conservatism from the 1950s: the tough love citizen recognized fraudulent bids for "special rights" and believed that middle-class life would be nice for everyone, but only if they earned it. Times were hard, but the tough love citizen could vote for the measures that dramatically expanded the underclass, even while they felt sorry for the homeless their detached compassion created.

The emergence of the new citizen was rather quick: the initial social response to the new epidemic was, it seems, widespread, if passive — sexphobia and panic toward gay men, drug injectors, homeless people, blacks, and sex workers. America capitalized on this initial response not by helping the needy, but by offering a new paradigm for citizenship: the compassionate, tolerant individual who, while never viewing him- or herself as susceptible to contracting HIV, could nevertheless recognize that "some of my best friends have HIV." Rock Hudson, Ryan White, Ali Geertz, Magic Johnson, and dozens of less extensively exposed local and national figures allowed compassionate citizens to form mediated relationships with people living with HIV. Alongside the citizens and their favorite "friend" were constructed not homosexuals or even queers, but deeply obscene bodies, densities that could be the object of research, treatment, discrimination, hatred, and even compassion, but that were inadmissible to the new body politic.

Thinking of these public information campaigns and media stories as a national pedagogy suggests that the idea of citizenship that pertained was not just an example of interpellation,[6] but evidence of a new procedure of subject formation, one in which the formal moments of "teaching" are only a part. America of the 1980s and 1990s is less the patriarchal, policing state imagined in Louis Althusser's classic example of the policeperson-citizen interaction than it is an avuncular nation of Bill Clintons and Ross Perots, who teach us what it means to be an American, of 20/20 and Moneyline, which teach us what an American is supposed to know and care about. For Althusser, power is structured domination by a state that protects class interests. Here, pedagogy's power arises through the invocation of a knowledge that simultaneously precedes and seamlessly becomes the possession of the hailed subject. For Althusser, education is just the state operating through less visibly violent ("ideologic") means. The complex interplay between medical and policy institutions and the forms of knowledge they produced highlighted the extent to which this nation does *not* exercise the form of control envisioned by Althusser: coming to think of ourselves is a much more fragile process. Thus, in the United States of the late 1980s, teaching the nation, threatening the citizen with stupidity rather than violence, is the central form of power: being an American requires extensive and overt lessons in politics, economy, world affairs, but most important, in cold compassion. The concept of national pedagogy suggests that power-knowledge is not *statically held* in a state comprised of both brute and sublime apparatuses, but is a *procedure* for bringing bodies into positions of duty and obligation that are constitutive of identity.[7]

Michel Foucault called various modes of relating bodies, space, and their administration "governmentalities." My main concern in this volume is the production and contestation of a particular form of governmentality — the national AIDS pedagogy. I want to suggest that if the state is more diffuse than activists of the 1980s imagined, then the efforts and effects of their projects must have been less clearly oppositional than neo-Marxian analysis suggested, less predictable than neopositive sociologies hoped. Power works differently than we had imagined; power is far more productive than our critiques of the 1980s recognized. Thus, instead of suggesting that the state "won" when it secured a national pedagogy, I will argue that the persistent contestation of that pedagogy through a variety of safe sex educational efforts coming from within gay communities (detailed in chapters 4 and 5) resulted in the constitution of two zones of information. Our contestations partially secured the national pedagogy (in a series of ways I will discuss in chapter 4), but (as chapters 3 and 5 will suggest) the national pedagogy also left open a space for dissident projects, but only by balkanizing the bodies whose safety depended on their ability to signify and ensure antinational practices of sex.

This jockeying founded the national pedagogy as a paradox: the gap between this new citizen and the dangerous bodies from which they were distinguished widened, even as average Americans were apparently increasingly concerned about the plight of people living with AIDS. Witness, for example, the way in which the red ribbon campaign so uneasily doubled the yellow ribbon campaign meant to demonstrate patriotism during the Gulf War, and how other ribbon colors have now proliferated as emblems of the citizen who cares deeply about victims (pink for breast cancer, purple for the people of Oklahoma City) but is ultimately unwilling to recognize or fund solutions. The sick within the national borders could be recognized as objects of American's compassion, but they could no longer fit into the ideal of citizenship. This paradox of separation and incorporation occurred through the slow production of a national pedagogy of AIDS, which attracted to itself systems of policing that rearticulated a "normal sexuality" in order to reterritorialize bodies that had gone ballistic in the 1960s and 1970s. The "sexual revolution" crashed in a heap, but citizens emerged from the wreck as self-consciously austere heterosexuals.

By the mid-1980s citizens could talk about AIDS, but only by desexualizing its vectors. Ill-disposed toward the antinational Me Generation and its pursuit of self and pleasure, citizens viewed the supposedly untrammeled hedonism of the 1970s as the "cause" of AIDS. But this sexuality existed only in allusion, as a past, as a "sexual revolution" that was hopefully now "over." Part of the compassion that would characterize the citizen came through romanticizing — "accepting" — the tragic flaw of the white, middle-class gay male professional "community" whose new-found pair bonding (" 'til death do us part") tacitly ensured an implosive end to the epidemic.

As the national pedagogy developed, gay communities responded to the AIDS epidemic and the representational crisis of the 1980s with multiple, conflicting forms of activism: the specific concern in this volume is the forms of political organizing that surrounded HIV prevention or "safe sex." These various projects, characterized in chapter 4, sometimes assimilated gay men to the sexual austerity that was increasingly a dimension of national identity, but sometimes rejected citizenship and refused the forms of information (especially advice to "just say no") through which the individual body was incorporated into the body politic. Safe sex organizing among gay men struggled over the same identity issues faced in the larger gay movement as it tried to negotiate its similarity to the citizen ("we're just like everyone else") but at the same time its need to spell out the difference that would mark minority status and make it possible to prove — and remedy — discrimination under civil rights provisions. Queer Nation would eventually try to circumvent debates between universalizing and minoritizing strategies[8] that troubled gay and AIDS activism of the 1980s. They proposed an alternate theory of national space that placed queerness as already and always present and *central* to Americanness. But the national pedagogy was one step ahead. From Arsenio Hall to departments of English to women's magazines' adoption of lesbian chic, mainstream America was braced for the more fashionable presentations of homoexoticism: the compassionate citizen was no longer offended by his/her proximity to queerness. She could maintain her difference and safety through the performance of kindness toward people living with AIDS, at least the now repentant sad men (as opposed to the angry ACT UP activists) who were enlisted to serve their country as objects of compassion.

Until the Surgeon General's 1988 campaign, there were no official, nation-wide efforts to promote risk reduction or even to explain clearly the mechanics of HIV transmission. Some might argue that the routes and proba- bilities of transmission were as yet unclear. The 1983 Callen and Berkowitz pamphlet "How to Have Sex in an Epidemic" refutes this contention. Pro- duced by several longtime gay activists in New York, "How to Have Sex" sorts through confusing data on the new epidemic and divergent theories of the syndrome's cause. Using their extensive knowledge about their own com- munity, Callen and Berkowitz offer what is still some of the best thinking about the epidemic and its meaning for gay men and produce a commonsense approach to practices and ethics. Importantly, these nonscientists produced advice that is still, for the most part, accurate.[9] Thus, during its formative years, the national pedagogy operated between the lines of a series of morality tales (beginning with Rock Hudson and ending with Magic Johnson) about America's "friend" who had AIDS. Although it disavowed any educational role, media circumlocution, together with government silence, taught the public how to understand and react to AIDS.

At first, fear of contagion spread like wild fire as random Americans engaged in truly despicable acts of hostility toward people associated with AIDS.[10] "America Responds to AIDS," the first national AIDS education campaign — the first articulate moment of a longer national AIDS pedagogy — was designed to quell fears about general contagion by enlightening the "ignorant" with "facts." Once educated, the citizen was expected to desist from the nastiest forms of discrimination, now considered unenlightened (individual terror was always exempt from criticism and law).[11] Compared to having to react to the phantasm of a Dark Ages–like plague, being nice to deviants was a breeze. Citizens heaved a collective sigh of relief and resolved to ensure their safety through the kinder, gentler posture of friend to the dying. But America was never really a kind or gentle place, so citizens needed to be reminded through ongoing lessons in compassion, opulently presented in human interest news features, fiction films, and made-for-television movies: NBC's movie *An Early Frost* (1985), NBC's news feature *Life, Death, and AIDS* (1986), the Public Broadcasting System's long-running AIDS *Quarterly* (1989–1991), the countless lyrical articles about the immune system and hard-nosed exposés of contemporary sexual mores, stories about volunteers (as opposed to "activists," also unpaid laborers in the epidemic), and, finally, relentlessly, the endless parables that put a "face" on AIDS by publicizing the lives and deaths of people living with HIV whose fifteen minutes of fame came at the cost of their privacy and, sometimes, safety.

This book extends several of my earlier essays[12] on AIDS education, which I wrote while I was actively engaged in developing safe sex projects. I undertook these revisions and reconsiderations in order to show how a national pedagogy was formed, how safe sex organizers coped with an evolving national project, and why they eventually turned to pornography as a means of representing and resignifying "safe" sex. This project seemed like an important first step in considering how what we learned in the 1980s can be of use in sexual liberation projects in the years ahead. Thus, a manifesto appears in place of a conclusion. The remainder of this chapter will provide a broad description of salient features of the 1980s, highlighting the genesis and logic of official educational programs. Chapter 2 will examine a single case of national pedagogy in action, detailing the media's construction of young people's risk for contracting HIV. Chapter 3 looks at the fatal collision of mainstream conceptions of adolescent innocence, as articulated through AIDS discourse, and a peculiar reading of pornography as documents proving the truth of an owner's sexual practice. Chapter 4 will describe the trajectory of gay community–based safe sex educational projects that sometimes collaborated in and sometimes contested national pedagogy. Chapter 5 takes up issues in the production of sexually explicit, even pornographic safe sex material. Finally, chapter 6 elaborates ways of understanding sexual vernacular as materially linked with space, a theory that, while it simultaneously reforms radical sexual politics, might also better support dissident pedagogies.

The Proliferation of Visible Desires

The movies, advertising, and pornography of the 1960s and 1970s were widely criticized by feminists and gay liberationists for not accurately representing their sexualities. But the grassroots productions designed to replace them did not fare much better. Gay men's sexual representations were nearly always commercialized, while lesbians' projects were almost never commercially viable.[13] And, despite the ambitions of gay and feminist-separatist culture producers and distributors of the 1970s, the political, technological, and social conditions of the 1980s changed so that virtually no self-representation could be totally protected from the voyeuristic, policing, or simply misinterpreting eye of the dominant culture. Heterosexual men marched into gay and feminist bookstores and bought things that had been produced by and for women or gay men. Or, the products simply slipped quietly beyond community borders — sometimes into Jerry Falwell's clutches, sometimes into the hands of uncomprehending wives, husbands, parents, or roommates, who inadvertently discovered suspicious items under the bed.

But it was not just the impossibility of protecting one's space that made "authentic voices" liable to violent appropriation or misreading: even the for-lesbians, by-lesbians magazines with tiny circulations did not find a homogenous or happy audience. Some women objected to particular images (especially S/M and bondage), but others believed sexual representation in itself always sullied a naturally unmediated sexuality. Bitter debates about the acceptability of representations of desire through "lesbian pornography" revealed that one woman's erotic fantasy of submission was another's documentation of patriarchal enslavement. These "sex wars" created huge fractures among lesbians, but these battles were fought largely outside the public eye.[14] Gay men's debates about their changing sexuality were similarly bitter — especially those concerning bathhouse closings or arrests of seropositive men accused of practicing unsafe sex. But because these conflicts also involved public health officials and were sensationalized in the mass media, they became deeply woven into the fabric of the national fantasy of the AIDS epidemic. Thus, *both* invisibility and overexposure created new ways through which sexuality was mediated and textualized.

In the 1980s, an epidemic of a strange new virus increased the sense of urgency to control sexuality, while the proliferation of remarkable forms of representing sexuality provided exemplary — to some, even frightening — objects to discuss. The virus was unusual in its slowness, taking as many as a dozen years to provoke palpable symptoms (although individuals may now preview their fate in the highly mediated event of HIV antibody testing). Those infected with HIV were *grounded,* linked by a series of proximate acts (sex, needle sharing, "the gift of life" received in transfusion of a stranger's blood, fetal-maternal symbiosis), "vectors" that comprised a tattered map of only dimly recalled physical contact. The new media, from music and cable television to home video, fax machines, and electronic mail, were remarkable for their speed and distortion of place. Computers and modems permitted us to "transmit" and receive information and images at astonishing speeds without ever leaving home. Juxtaposed as extremes of speed and slowness, proximity and displacement, the media and the virus nevertheless served as mutual metaphors: scientists talked about messenger RNA and remarked that the virus was "trying to tell us something." Hastened along by postmodern cultural critics, the decay of reassuring metanarratives — for example, the transparency of communication — was likened to RNA-DNA replication and its dangerous errors: for minimalist musician Laurie Anderson (1985) "language [was] a virus."

A late-twentieth-century version of Nietzsche's army of mobile metaphors connected the virus and the media, and tore us away from the mundane, everyday reality of bodies, of *our* bodies. We began to pursue our lives in the hyperspace — hypospace? — vacated by the body. We had more "information" than we knew what to do with, and, yet, we seemed completely incapable of seeing ourselves except through truncated mirrored glances. Void and surfaceless, the human-scale body so necessary for understanding and incorporating risk-reducing sexual techniques met a blank screen when it came to sex. Ideas about safe sex were cacophonous, yet there were few opportunities to actually *learn* what it looked and felt like, much less how to *do* it.

Euro-American culture alternately considered sexuality frivolous or unspeakable, bawdy or inarticulate. The imprecision and polyvalence of the language of sex had been a source of humor: it was "hard" to know when we were talking about sex and when we were talking about business or politics or other weighty matters. The appearance of sexology in the late 1800s had to some extent robbed Euro-Americans' sexual languages of their metaphoric flexibility: scientists pressed the utterances of sexualities into a more precise language *about* sex. Dissident sexual vernaculars publicly returned in the flagrant 1960s and 1970s as the women's sexual freedom and gay liberation movements produced no-holds-barred texts that demoted the penis, debated the forms of female orgasm, and suggested that real men "take it," too. The underground pornographies of working-class homosexuals, male desire for female domination, and sexes made equal by the desire for raw visual slime howled at the edges of mainstream media institutions. "Art films" and hard core porn converged in cinematic style; *Blue Boy* made its way to the convenience store rack next to *Playboy;* and feminist magazines and books liberated women's desires to be dominated and to dominate — desktop-published, grassroots erotica began to compete with the mass market romance novels that served up female desires in less overtly political terms.

The language of sex and the contexts in which it was deemed appropriate to speak of sex were radically fractured and fragmented. We could apparently speak more frankly than ever before, although the New Right was making apocalyptic predictions about the consequences of all this talking. And there was not, as popularly suggested, an inverse relation between talking about sex and doing it. No indeed. In the 1980s, text and sex merged: the line between reading a sexual text and *being* a sexual text was blurred. Americans were a tribe textually constructed through our love of one-hand reads: we were pornographic, masturbatory.

In addition to new populist narratives of sexual desire, clinical studies by sexologists told us what our neighbors were donig. A range of typically American how-to books promised to improve our technique. The disciplinary erotics of clinical description and the sheer antiromanticism of Kegel exercises provided a new language about sex that disavowed desire, even as it incited fetishistic — or perhaps sadomasochistic — pleasure in the mechanized body observed and improved.

Increased economic and social power for some women reopened discus-

Around 1989
———

sion of bi- and homosexualities, highlighting the realities of sexual competition in a widening market. The recognition of the demands of female pleasure (along with the admission that traditional coitus was technically deficient — or, to put it more bluntly, that dinky penises were insufficient to produce female orgasm through intercourse) recast sex from the transcendent *jouissance* of pair bonding to a play of parallel and mutually incomprehensible *plaisirs*. Performance anxiety, and the technical how-to manuals that tried to quell it, formed a new kind of erotic literature that replaced the lushly illustrated and mystically descriptive books of karma sutra variations once popular with the free-love generation. Sex was drawn under the careful regression analyses of demographers who deciphered the shifts in market forces won through decreasing penalties for racial, gender, and sexual difference. On the individual level, Kinsey statistics replaced Casanova-like tales as benchmarks of sexual conquest. The local video store stocked a new style of pornography to view at home, and soon one could buy "home" porn videos by/of "ordinary people" having "ordinary" sex. The appearance of real penises and vaginas, complete with wrinkles and wayward pubic hairs (and bad camera angles), created a documentary aura around even the most fantastically improbable sex. The narrative structure of the new pornography satisfied the lust for realism that Hollywood refused to accommodate.

It is, of course, now analytically forbidden to conclude that there was a sudden release from a "repression." But the transformation of sex into overt and self-reflexive texts not immediately tied to activities culturally designated as "sex" seemed to reach a new level of undeniability. If, as Foucault (1972) suggested, a fundamental template provides the conditions for what can be authoritatively said in an era, then the proliferation of texts that has flattened meaning and that has characterized postmodernity finally broke a basic "statement" of the modern sexual episteme. The barrage of texts — from pornography to science to how-to books and magazine columns — that made truth claims about sex evacuated any lingering pretense that there was a fixed essence in sexuality. Sex lost its reality, its ability to rally the support of a fully dominant form of practice — and gender came tumbling after. If penile-vaginal intercourse was still in vogue, it was challenged from several fronts as it sought to reliably convey the mantle of safety that heterosexual identity was supposed to afford.

New technologies arrived at an ominous time. While it seems clear that Reaganism brought a massive challenge to the antiracist, antisexist, and anti-homophobic efforts of the previous two decades, gender and sexuality became destabilized in ways that cannot be fully captured through the idea of backlash. Alongside the glosses that the spin doctors daubed onto the Great Communicator were major changes in mainstream and alternative media production and consumption. The proliferation of home video and cable television and the narrow casting these made possible conspired with the economic recession to produce a "stay at home" ethos that forced men and women to consume, learn the interpretive regimes and codes of, complain about, and feel embarrassed by genres whose consumption had once been gender segregated.

New technologies radically altered the modes of producing and consuming alternative media, democratizing production through decreasing the cost of, in particular, video and magazine production. The Hi-8 video camera and desktop publishing enabled relatively small groups of people to produce and circulate images, polemics, and theory of/for themselves. But as the movement of countermedia blossomed, the mainstream media against which it chafed also changed, as did the theoretical understanding of relations among production, consumption, and interpretation. Although some theorists clung to a traditional hypodermic model[15] in which messages and images were metaphorically injected into a largely passive audience, those most actively involved in producing and consuming the new countermedia were forced to recognize that neither they, nor the people with/for whom they produced their work, engaged in predictable interpretive practices. Mass market producers could no longer assume that traditional genres would be legible to new audiences, and countercultural producers could no longer be sure that their disruption of "stereotypes" would be read through an oppositional political consensus.

The sharpest area of contention was, of course, in the arena of representations of sex and sexuality. The urgency of the AIDS epidemic provided the impetus for rapid and aggressive national intervention into the sexual lives and symbolic systems of Americans. But with a few tragic exceptions, the state was disinclined to intervene too brutally or explicitly. Instead, the media and government agencies unwittingly embarked on a campaign to reframe the meaning of sex and, especially, to wrest control over the concept of *safe* sex.

Around 1989

17

The prerogative to apply names is one of the most contended forms of power in the late twentieth century. Disenfranchised groups of the 1960s and 1970s had high hopes for the names and concepts they forged for themselves. But the polyphony of differences among Americans became muted in the 1980s as a national AIDS pedagogy proposed a new, unified form of citizenship that was held open to anyone, but attainable only by those who were already part of the 1950s dream of normalcy. The 1980s and 1990s are a sobering object lesson in the relatively greater power held by science, government, and media to name, rename, and take over the names groups make for themselves. AIDS organizers and activists, especially, learned a hard lesson: it is difficult to predict the results of discursive battles. But this was not just a problem of securing activists' meanings; their ideas were taken up and modified by officials, rendering activism partially successful, but without affording activists any stable base of power. Radical critique could no longer just "tell it like it is" in order to rip the scales of ideology from people's eyes; critique was complexly enmeshed in the process of constructing and reconstructing discursive and institutional power.

The naming of the epidemic provides an easy example of the dynamics of this process. "AIDS" maintained its ideological connection with Western gay men through three changes in nomenclature — Gay Related Immune Deficiency, Acquired Immune Deficiency Syndrome, Human Immunodeficiency Virus disease — which reflected different understandings of the relation between bodies and disease. Activists' accusations of homophobia, along with the scientific recognition of substantial numbers of AIDS cases among people who were not gay men, prompted the change from GRID to AIDS. Activists next criticized the use of AIDS — the probably fatal late stage of a longer, chronic viral process — as the name for the viral process as a whole. They believed the connotative value of AIDS as a "death sentence" promoted a fatalism that was psychologically harmful to those who had the virus. Many scientists agreed that AIDS was a problematic name, but for reasons of their own: terms like "HIV spectrum" or "HIV disease" not only reflected their narrative about the course of the virus, but also rationalized the varying levels of medical intervention (antivirals trials, and later, experimental high-technology treatments like bone marrow transplants) to which they hoped those who had contracted the virus might wish to submit at different "stages."

But despite these challenges and changes, the AIDS-gay connection held fast. The activist-scientist struggle over names was only the most superficial level of a whole range of namings that stemmed from the deep — and con-tinuing — association of the medical phenomenon with a group of people thought to have a unique trait that marked them as deviant. "GRID" suggested that pathology lay in something "gay-related": the syndrome was synony-mous with those who had it. But "AIDS" tapped into another complicated cultural discourse: "choosing" to be "gay" was easily equated with "acquir-ing" "immunodeficiency." Even the "spectrum" of "HIV disease" con-formed to one trajectory of modern Western beliefs about sexuality: from Freudian psychology to Queer Nation's explosion of narrow ideas of gay identity to Roseanne's response to her lesbian kiss,[16] one popular under-standing of sexuality has been that most people are at least a little queer. But even this persistent idea did not end homophobia or provide a rationale to explain why "anyone" could "get AIDS." Instead, the idea of polymorphous perversity suggested that securing one's heterosexuality was in itself a form of safe sex.

The AIDS-gay association that has shaped activism, policy, representation, and research is more than a tragic example of deeply entrenched homophobia. In fact, a whole range of ideas — challenged and enlisted by activists — stem from this early codification. These ideas, which arose from activist-scientist skirmishes, are now central to government policy and to the representations that frame compassionate citizenship. They sometimes serve as a lever for activism, but sometimes they split activists along lines of gender and race. In particular, gay people's assertion of themselves as a community has helped define what the body politic *is:* it is *not* a community. The citizen possesses a national, not an individual, identity, while their Other — especially the gay person — *is* totally subsumed by the elements that make them different, by their identification with that difference. The citizen *has* traits like heterosex-ual, family-oriented, etc., but is identified by their tolerant disposition toward people associated with AIDS. Thus, the voice and visibility for which gay activists of the 1970s fought became the very criteria for barring them from citizenship; by the 1980s, the citizen was ordinary, not identifiable, unarticulated, "everybody else." Gay community was confused with "risk group": the "general public" seemed to think the entire gay community was "at risk," and not from homophobia, as activists argued, but from their sexual practices.

The speed and strength of gay men's responses also made it clear that there *were* gay communities, many of which also included lesbians and other people whose sexualities did not fit comfortably within the mainstream. These collective responses afforded organized gay communities (primarily in the Northern European countries, the United States, Canada, and Australia) some power in shaping their nations' AIDS policies. Through extensive debate about and involvement in early epidemiologic studies, men who claimed gay identities were partially successful at dislinking identity from sexual acts. Researchers could focus on specific, clear routes of transmission, and activists could build on a positive definition of gay sexuality as organized around and as comprised of activities that were already and still "safe."

But because risk was associated with a subculture, few risk reduction or health education efforts emerged from the U.S. public health offices until 1986. Then, when it appeared that heterosexuals could become infected with HIV, the "public" was converted into a "community." Because identity and practices had been collapsed in media accounts about AIDS it was easy to transform "heterosexuality" into a default identity. The hysterical admonitions that "anyone can get AIDS" really meant that you can't tell who is bisexual by looking. The initial confusion between identities and acts re-emerged to provide a corollary "safe" space for non-gay people. Men with a gay identity were all presumed to engage in specific, "risky," homosexual acts. The absence of those acts in others conveyed to them a heterosexual identity. The strong connotative meanings of identity and community had changed. Identity was no longer oppositional — "not straight" — and community no longer marked subcultural affinity. By the end of the 1980s, when researchers and the media spoke about non-gay, sexually active people who might be at risk of contracting HIV, they replaced "public" or "mainstream" with the phrase "heterosexual community." But the "heterosexual community" was a simulacrum produced through epidemiology and the media: it lacked the social reality, the sensibility of the "gay community," which, through decades of defending its members against homophobia, had forged common interests and values and now shared resources like alternative media, businesses, and clinics. To the extent that risk reduction information would always emerge from or be targeted at "communities," the lack of shared norms and sensibilities of the "heterosexual community" would render "safe sex" unreal.

In place of a mobilizable sexual identity, the national pedagogy promoted general identification with the idea of the compassionate citizen. This figure emerged in opposition to the connotations of "identity" and "community" that were related to urban gay men's experience of and activism in the epidemic. This new public, carved out of the people against whom gay people once marked their difference, was now itself constructed oppositionally: *not at risk of contracting* HIV. An asymmetry of oppositions was now stabilized, and these became the central terms through which the epidemic was — is — understood: gay equals not straight, citizen equals not at risk, not at risk equals compassionate, not compassionate equals potential sex monster. The very concepts of identity and community that had been consolidated through U.S. gay men's efforts to reorganize their collective sexual practice in the context of the diffuse and contradictory representations of "safe sex" were now the very mechanism that made it possible to prevent them from being citizens. The national pedagogy initially depended on a consensus about who was "abnormal." But the vague heterosexual, white, middle-class, nonaddicted, etc., bodies that had once simply been "everyone else" in relation to the deviations and minorities was soon more clearly marked as the *citizen.* The national pedagogy finally enabled the sociological "norm" to take up a place in the late twentieth century's most extensive discourse of the body.

In this dynamic and ongoing process of framing and reframing, categories of political visibility partially insinuated gay men's ideas of themselves into the research/policy/media enterprise. But this also resulted in a significant loss of control over the terms used to stage activism, with significant repercussions for gay men. How do we deal with "men who have sex with men"? Ease them toward "gay identity" or be "culturally sensitive" and let them practice *ex nominalis?* The facility with which gay men could now speak in the same terms as these powerful institutions also affected their capacity to form activist coalitions across the categories epidemiology and the media proposed and naturalized: between gay men and women, between gay men and people of color, between gay men and drug injectors (presumed to be straight) whose risk was not thought to derive from sexual behaviors.

But perhaps most damaging, as the idea of a "heterosexual community"

Around 1989

21

took hold, the oppositional form and historical place of gay community began to fade from view, especially for younger gay people, who must have seen "community" as a neutral descriptor of each of two "lifestyle" "choices." This shift in the meaning of community suggested that oppression arose from individuals' AIDS-phobia, not systemic heterosexism, reframing the task of community organizing from the liberationist form it had taken in early AIDS activism. Many gay men's energies were now directed toward reeducating the public, not about gay life, but about how "You can't get AIDS from a door-knob." Instead of helping individuals recognize their own relationship to and possible membership in gay community, indeed, instead of describing the fluidity of sexuality, educators conveyed the "facts about AIDS" without cultivating a memory of queer resistance. Young men who entered gay worlds in the 1980s knew more about retrovirology than they did about the history of the communities they joined. Rarely did these young men challenge the stories they read in the national media: they, too, interpreted gay liberation as a simple, even selfish libertinism, the cause of the epidemic's proliferation rather than a historic source of collective power to mobilize against political backlash.

When the media — and its young gay readers — displaced the responsibility for the effects of homophobia onto gay culture or gay liberation, they undermined the strength and the values that gay communities had honed through decades of resisting social policing. Even safe sex educators adopted the revisionist history over the oppositional memory: they viewed both the supposed sexual license of the 1970s and the response to AIDS as exceptional. Because they were reluctant to ground their programs in a historical critique of the social and medical control of sexuality, they jeopardized the scope and durability of their calls to safe sex. As long as the "cause" of AIDS was situated in unusual circumstances of unusual individuals, the structural and systemic forces that impeded large-scale changes in sexual, medical, and discriminatory practices would remain unchallenged. On the individual level, this made safe sex appear as punishment for antisocial deeds committed by libertines in the past: even for gay men, this suggested that the politically astute position was limitations on sexuality. Few activists were able to rally support for the claim that safe sex was a new form of fighting back, an honorable inheritor of survival strategies that had been developed through years of fighting queer bashing, psychological terrorism (lobotomy, aversion therapy, institutionalization), medical indifference (no research on special health needs, no preventative or primary care for STDS), police harassment, job and housing discrimination, and ridicule.

As we will see in the Savitz case (chapter 3), safe sex, stripped of the collective memory of earlier forms of homosexual repression and viewed as a penalty, reopened parts of the gay community to the same kinds of psychological and social policing that characterized the U.S. government's early response to the HIV epidemic. The gay community's general failure to conceptualize changing norms as an intracommunity project left warring groups of gay men to blame each other for stretching the boundaries of sexual experimentation. This tension underscored the development of increasingly distinct projects, some undertaken by health education traditionalists within the gay community who wrested funds from government agencies, and some pursued more organically by dissident safe sex organizers who had more of a grounding in representation theory than in health education pedagogy.

There is no way to ultimately resolve the tension between the "mainstream" and "community" understandings of "safe sex," since official nominating bodies — media, government agencies, research and policy enterprises — finally have more power to disperse meanings. The remainder of this chapter will describe how broad-based, supposedly apolitical health education strategies became the means for dividing educational subjects into those who would be formed into citizens through a national pedagogy and those who would be policed or, if they were lucky, ignored as they developed their own dissident safe sex strategies.

Health Education: Risk versus Population

Health educators from within and outside the "risk" communities have grounded their projects in a variety of theories; however, these generally have grown out of one of two broad paradigms, one based on decreasing risk by modifying the behavior of an entire population, and one based on decreasing risk by targeting only those believed to be at highest risk. Although, in practice, AIDS prevention programs from different paradigms have often occurred simultaneously,[17] most programs have been designed with one paradigm in mind. Selection of these health education strategies has depended on subtle differences in the perception of a disease phenomenon, generally: (1) the epidemiologic perception of the degree of emergency posed by a health phenomenon; (2) the popular and health establishment's perception of the odiousness of the change or precaution advocated; and, importantly, though less often acknowledged, (3) general social perceptions of and attitudes toward those believed to be subject to a disorder. Both the population-based and risk-based approaches have recognized that individuals would be differentially affected by both the disease syndrome and the sought-after change, but they have differed in *how* they have maximized disease prevention.

The population-wide strategy has viewed risk as a continuum and assumed that many people were at some level of risk. An aggregate, population-wide decrease in the dangerous behavior or condition would also then result in a decrease among those most at risk. Population-based programs have perceived the health precaution or change to be beneficial for everyone, harmful to no one, and relatively simple and nonoffensive to adopt. By contrast, risk-focused strategies have attempted to alert particular types of people to their special risk. Risk has been viewed as virtually absolute: one either is or isn't at risk. In addition, the proposed change in sexual practices has been viewed as unfairly restrictive or burdensome or simply not useful enough to impose on those not clearly at risk.

As I will suggest here, the two trajectories of AIDS education of the 1980s targeted ideologically opposed audiences and differed in strategic form. Because epidemiologists perceived that AIDS signaled an extreme emergency and that homosexuals and drug injectors were geographically isolated and extremely deviant, and because heterosexuals demonstrated a distaste for condoms and were disinclined to experiment with alternatives to intercourse, prevention campaigns were locked into risk-based, rather than population-based, programming. In contrast to these targeted risk-reduction campaigns, the national pedagogy, which suggested that there was very little cost in giving up discriminatory attitudes, embarked on a population-wide campaign to quell fears of mass contagion and to promote compassion toward people living with AIDS (compassion towards the merely infected was always contingent on proof that they were containing the epidemic).[18]

The split in AIDS education complicated the official response, especially in the increasingly conservative 1980s. The trick was to construct a nationally controlled pedagogy that did not require a population-wide sexual health campaign. The initial solution was to say very little about the emerging epidemic. But this general reticence was more insidious than the usual descriptions of a media blackout on AIDS information suggest. While the gross *amount* of news coverage was small compared to what was to come, the *content* was quite sensational: whatever stories there were stuck in readers' minds. Despite AIDS beat reporters' contention that their role was to inform, not to "educate," the media formed the most basic element of the national pedagogy, constructing readers' concerns and providing a framework for the ensuing avalanche of information.

The media reported AIDS information in two ways: as science, reported as breaking news, and through prevention advice, conveyed through oblique allusions to how or why famous or stereotypical people became infected. The latter, morality tale-cum-gossip format was refined through coverage of Ryan White's life and death and reached its apotheosis in the coverage of Magic Johnson's life after his discovery that he was seropositive. Both White and Johnson were produced as the special friend of the compassionate citizen who could now know about, but who would never engage in, the sordid activities that might allow HIV transmission. Although they rarely expressly advocate safe sex, these accounts produced an interpretive framework through which citizens could learn about routes of transmission without actually imagining that this information might apply to themselves. Both coverage *about* AIDS science and interchangeable stories featuring people living with HIV encouraged readers to take up an observer's position, rather than to view themselves as the bodies under discussion: the potentially infected body became the object of the citizen's voyeurism.

Whatever objective tone they adopted, the media were far from neutral. Even when their content was dry and scientific, the media subtly reinforced the safety and distance of the citizen. Scientific breakthroughs were rarely described as of specific benefit to the reader: people living with HIV might be quoted as "hopeful," but the primary message was that science was in control, and that the epidemic would indeed not extend beyond the presently affected demographic groups. The persistent representation of "new drugs" as "cures," and the generality of explanation about them, suggested that the

Around 1989

reader was not really interested in exactly how a drug worked, or in precisely which opportunistic infections it might treat, or in relation to which theory of HIV progression the drug had meaning. At least through the 1980s, the media used evocative but less specific scientific terms ("natural killer" and "helper" cells, rather than specifying the cell name as it would have appeared in the reported research or on an individual's laboratory tests), patronizingly distinguished between HIV and AIDS[19] (as if the reader might not know this), valorized minute virologic breakthroughs with little immediate use, or underplayed the development of treatments for opportunistic infections, the "medicine" that had real effects on people's lives. Apparently, the reader was not infected, not interested in the details of research because it did not directly affect their quality of life.

Separate Spheres, Opposite Strategies

As soon as the emerging syndrome was linked with a perceived subgroup, homosexuals, AIDS epidemiology and educational efforts generated from the Public Health Service employed a risk-based approach. Rapidly changing social attitudes about sexuality and drug use rendered the notion of risk groups highly equivocal because it referred to subcultures that were already labeled socially deviant and were presumed to be virtually autonomous from the perceived mainstream population. Ironically, gay people's battles to reclaim once stigmatized social labels as positive cultural identities meant that there was an uncomfortable convergence between groups' hard-won notions of community and epidemiologists' labeling of risk groups. Despite efforts among activists to shift terminology from risk group to risk behavior, AIDS education information concerning risk *reduction* was directed almost exclusively toward gay men, and soon (though much less consistently) toward injection drug users.

Although public health officials advocated use of a risk-based approach, the federal and most state governments did not back up their strategy with funding. Right-wing watchdogs insisted that promoting new (or sustaining existing), low-risk ways to engage in stigmatized sexual and drug practices would increase deviant behavior: this perception was made into national law with the passage of the Helms Amendment.[20] In a climate of increasing social conservatism, the decision by public health officials to use a risk-based approach meant that relatively little government-sponsored risk reduction information would ever be produced or distributed. Education for those "at risk" was considered obscene and immoral, and risk reduction was considered unnecessary for anyone else. With the exception of the Centers for Disease Control Demonstration Projects, which survived largely by using complicated terminology ("men who have sex with men," "people who exchange sex for money or drugs," "hard to reach populations") and by putting the restrictions on use of explicit material in fine print, the vast majority of the 1980s safe sex campaigns directed toward gay men were funded through private sources, usually individual donations from members of the gay community, and later through the independent American Foundation for AIDS Research (AmFAR).

By the mid-1980s, it was evident that the "general public" had problematic misperceptions about AIDS, especially regarding the feasibility of casual transmission. The public health service responded with a population-based educational campaign aimed at the "general public," designed to explain the specificity of modes of HIV transmission and to attack discrimination.[21] This effort culminated in the controversial 1988 Surgeon General's report, which largely assumed that while risk reduction knowledge was nice, the general population, never imaged to be at risk, should be educated mainly about the impossibility of contracting HIV through casual or social contact. In the immediate context of hysteria, federally supported pleas for compassion toward people living with AIDS helped provide a more positive atmosphere for the legal battles of the mid-1980s. HIV was classified as a perceived handicap, enabling people with HIV to claim discrimination under existing disability laws. In some cases, HIV was specifically included in city antidiscrimination codes. But in the longer term, the Surgeon General's report cemented the split between those perceived to be at risk — who still received no official risk reduction advice — and the "general public," who were now wiser, if not always nicer.

By the late 1980s, not only were there two different kinds of AIDS education campaigns under way, targeting audiences through two different strategies, but the messages they conveyed were actually contradictory if applied to a single person: one could not be compassionate toward potentially in-

Around 1989

fected Others and recognize oneself as potentially infected at the same time. Surrounded (at least in their community media) by people much like themselves who were infected, gay men managed to bridge this gap through a selfless, but regretful, heroism, whose image was the dying man's Buddy who was himself infected. Seropositive women were at the other extreme: able to recognize and project maternal compassion toward her infected child while still only dimly recognizing that she, too, had been infected by her male partner. Although education was widely spoken of as the epidemic's "only vaccine," risk was highlighted more than risk reduction, and no one was really encouraged to take up safe sex or safe drug use behaviors.

Thus, by the late 1980s, the contradictory AIDS education campaigns promulgated two forms of fatal advice, one of which downplayed the need to think about sexual behavior, while the other practically goaded individuals to imagine the one act that was produced as most dangerous. In one breath, the national pedagogy discouraged the general public from worrying about safe sex as long as they engaged in "ordinary" intercourse: their call to consciousness was simply to be nice to people with AIDS. In the next breath, they told gay men to believe that engaging in intercourse was the central and defining feature of their sexuality, but an activity from which it was now essential to desist.

This split in educational efforts resulted in a quite dramatic and literal difference in the density of information available in the "general" and "subcultural" spheres. The very lack of risk reduction information available in the public sphere may have actually reinforced citizens' belief in their lack of risk ("if it was important, they'd tell me about it"). Similarly, the sheer density and multivocality of information produced by gay men — at least within the urban core — probably contributed to a belief that risk reduction was important, even if not everyone always engaged in it.

In addition to different densities of information, different personal strategies for risk reduction were proposed for the two domains. In the national public, where lessons in risk reduction were few and far between, the citizen was encouraged to view risk as remote and to use avoidance tactics: "Choose your partner carefully." In a section called "What about Dating?" the 1980s' most widely distributed campaign to the general public (Surgeon General's Report 1988) contained this advice:

Fatal Advice
———
28

You are going to have to be careful about the person you become sexually involved with, making your own decision based on your own best judgement. That can be difficult.

Has this person had any sexually transmitted diseases? How many people have they been to bed with? Have they experimented with drugs? All these are sensitive, but important, questions. But you have a personal responsibility to ask. (4)

There were no details about how to effect such an interrogation: sex became an embarrassing and odious task, not an opportunity for erotic discovery. Partner avoidance was a personal, even private, responsibility, not a community-building project.

By contrast, the initial information produced within the gay communities, crisscrossed with advice in gay newspapers, pamphlets, and talks, encouraged a universal precaution strategy. Men should practice safe sex regardless of their or their partners' serostatus or probable past exposure to HIV: everyone should adopt routine use of condoms or simply avoid intercourse. The introduction to the Gay Health Action Group of Dublin safe sex pamphlet (1989) is especially articulate but does not differ from its American cousins in its concern to promote universal precautions rather than the partner selection strategy:

The "AIDS Crisis" does *not* mean that sex is a thing of the past. Sex can be safe. Much of what gay men have always done together has been "safe," and has no risk of passing the AIDS virus. It's simple to learn what's safe and what isn't.

Safer sex doesn't mean that we have to "stick to one partner," or be afraid to start up with a new lover. . . . What matters is that we don't transmit the virus. (2)

Like many community-based campaigns, this one emphasized the continuity between the new concept of safe sex and already and always safe practices inherited from gay culture of the preepidemic years. Safe sex knowledge was presented as simple to understand, not a mind-boggling medical menu, but a plan based on the bottom-line edict of nontransmission.

The don't-ask-don't-tell strategy adopted by many gay men who em-ployed — and still employ–universal safe sex was initially intended to avoid losing control over information that could result in legal discrimination.[22] But it also challenged the interrogative mode of the national pedagogy, which incited speech in private but banned sexually explicit talk in public. Like the vast networks of informers in the former Eastern bloc countries, good citizens performed a task that the government was loathe to directly organize. The good citizen was to investigate their partner's sexual past but not speak of sex too publicly. By contrast, the universal safe sex strategy engendered vociferous and often provocative public discussion of sex in order to ensure that individual compliance did not *require* extensive private discussion.

Prevention education was still persistently and insidiously linked with surveillance. While there was no central registry of those suspected or admitted to be HIV seropositive, sexual rejection became a quieter form of national witch-hunt. But even though citizens were learning that it was their "personal responsibility to ask" about their partners' actual or probable serostatus, the Public Health Service could not resist the temptation to more formally and publicly identify seropositives. Outside gay communities, acquiring detailed information about safe sex was increasingly contingent on one's attending the proliferating HIV antibody testing centers: tragically, the overinvestment in testing meant that the price of learning about safe sex was knowledge that one was already infected.

Testing the Nation

The first federal funding for education in communities became available in late 1985 and came with restrictions, including potential censorship by a "community standards" board and a requirement that education be linked to the then-new antibody test and its emerging counseling protocols. If education programs were not located at testing centers, then they were required to encourage participants to seek testing. Apparently the Public Health Service saw community education as partly social marketing of safe sex and partly an advertisement for testing. This funding pattern conflated surveillance and prevention and shaped the direction of safe sex programs that sought government funding.[23]

Originally, epidemiologists envisioned testing as the means to verify their theory that AIDS was caused by a sexually transmitted virus and to halt transmission by discovering who among those at risk was actually infected. Almost immediately upon licensure, HIV antibody testing became the centerpiece of the national plan to contain HIV. As early as the 1985 International Conference on AIDS in Atlanta, held before testing centers were officially implemented, the CDC's Donald Francis presented a mathematical model that purported to show how the new epidemic could be stemmed if all "gay men" were tested and had sex only with men of like antibody status. Francis's proposal treated gay male sexual culture like a giant dating service where serostatus (rather than love, desire, or common hobbies) would be the chief determinant of compatibility. This idea imposed on gay men the precise logic rejected by activists of the universal precautions school; indeed, this rational selection model would soon be revamped to become the central feature of the citizen's safe sex plan: avoiding sex with potentially seropositive individuals. Francis's model ignored the hazards to the already infected of reinfection or coinfection with other sexually transmitted pathogens and took little account of the many men (perhaps the majority) who had sex with men but who did not consider themselves "gay." But the CDC's panic at losing control of AIDS education to dissident projects was most evident in Francis's dismissal of the shift toward safe sex, already evident among urban gay men.

From 1985 on, national AIDS funding packages assumed that knowledge of antibody status would result in and reinforce behavioral changes. No data were yet available to support this view, and health education wisdom was divided on the general effectiveness of confrontational styles of education. The original testing mandates were, in effect, an experiment in social engineering and seemed only haphazardly and temporarily effective at producing individual behavior change. Having scoffed at safe sex techniques and having been encouraged to develop ever more complex systems of partner selection, heterosexuals jumped on testing as the ultimate means of clearing potential mates. Despite ad campaigns that told citizens that you "can't tell" who might be infected, they continued to rely on individual theories of who was potentially infected. HIV antibody testing now seemed to provide the answer to achieving risk elimination: an external way to verify their personal selection schemes. The very presence of testing and its interpretation as arbiter of the need to practice safe sex provided a veneer of scientific validity for capricious partner selection strategies. Citizens concluded that because, in principle, you could *know,* you could also develop educated guesses about whether someone was more likely to tell you what they knew or to lie. Some circumvented the testing process while referencing the knowledge that might have been obtained: they used fatal lore about who might be *un*infected as if it stood in for a negative test result.[24]

Around 1989
———————

31

Gay men of the universal precautions school urged men to simply imagine that anyone and everyone might be infected, and emphasized that a negative test was only valid if the last occasion of potential exposure was six months or a year earlier.[25] Few gay men knew about Francis's plan, and now that testing was a big topic on citizens' and the media's lips, gay men in large numbers thought they were being offered an alternative to the condom.

Recognizing the technical problems with testing and the likelihood that gay men, at least over a lifetime, would change partners, gay community groups clung to their well-honed and at least partially effective advocacy of universal safe sex. Dissident projects now had to counter the national pedagogy's proposition that testing was the simple solution to the sex problem of the 1980s. The following advice from the New York Gay Men's Health Crisis pamphlet about HIV antibody testing (1989) walks the reader through the logic of using testing in partner selection, but finally advocates condom use as the *easiest* program for a lifetime commitment to safer sex, even for those in monogamous couples who test seronegative:

Should I take the test so that I can stop practicing safer sex? If you and your partner use the test for this purpose, you both must remain absolutely monogamous, and continue to practice safer sex for at least a year before taking the test. This will ensure accuracy.

If you are both HIV-negative, and stop practicing safer sex, you and your partner must continue to be absolutely monogamous. Unprotected sex with even one person may expose you and your partner to HIV infection. To avoid this risk, it is safest simply to continue practicing safer sex, even if you think that you are in a monogamous relationship.

The difference between the gay community's increasing dissidence and the national pedagogy's insistence that citizens can simply avoid suspect partners is even clearer if we compare the above GMHC pamphlet to a concurrent pamphlet produced by the City of New York (1989) entitled "For men who have sex with men" (significantly, represented as African American), a phrase commonly used in campaigns aimed at men outside the information-dense gay communities: "Here's what you can do: If there is any chance that you or your partner might have the virus, use latex condoms (rubbers) whenever you have sex with another man or a woman." Even if straight-identified "men who have sex with men" succeed in recognizing themselves as the subjects addressed in this pamphlet, making condom use contingent on perceptions of infection — "if" — triggers the logic of the avoidance strategy.

By the 1990s, the very meaning of HIV testing depended on individuals' and communities' perceptions of their own risk. The early linkage between testing and prevention was built on top of, and served as a means of placing individuals within, differing spheres of safe sex knowledge and practice. Even the languages of sexuality served to distinguish between the two spheres. The citizen, at least in public, increasingly spoke of his/her sexuality in formal, homogeneous, and deeroticized terms. The official national language of safe sex did not include requests for hot rubber or jimmy caps. For gay men, who recognized their strange collective fate as subject of a medical phenomenon, and who believed they might contract HIV, testing promised access to prophylactic treatments or clinical trials.[26] But for citizens, HIV continued to be unreal, principally a frightening new example of the age-old hazards of unconventional sex, a fear that their compassion increasingly quelled. Citizens learned to confess or extract details of each other's sex lives and submitted to counseling and testing sessions that taught them how to ask and tell their sexual histories. "The test," erroneously and fatally enough, was their mechanism for determining whether to use condoms with a specific partner or to discover whether past partner selection strategies had been adequate.

The Next Generation

The two worlds of AIDS education created new conditions for policing sexuality by enunciating different educational subjects with different reasons to learn about AIDS. The first were members of the communities that had been begrudgingly allowed to speak frankly if they kept their dirty little secret to themselves. They needed to know how to protect themselves from HIV and each other. The citizen needed to learn compassion for people living with HIV, but not *so* much compassion that they ceased their vigilant efforts to "choose carefully" with whom they would have sex. Once honed, this exact split underwrote education for youth.

National pedagogy, as Frank (1995) has argued, is nowhere more evident and poignant than when directed toward the emerging citizen. But as certain as the nation is that it *must* educate, what and how were, through the 1980s, increasingly contentious. Between the "PC" debates, presidential round-tables, and violence in the schools, the process and practice of educating America's youth became a national crisis. Debates about education were most volatile and had the most immediate consequences when they concerned the sexualities of youth: the nation strained to create a path from the innocence of one family to the safety of another. But Reaganite fantasies had little to do with the lives and practices of most youth, who trod the same paths as the adults in the communities from which they came or, for gay youth, from which they fled. The 1989 WHO-GPA World AIDS Day had focused on youth, but citizens were more comfortable pitying street children in Brazil or orphans in Africa than offering their own children a means to survive the increasingly proximate epidemic.

In 1990, epidemiologists acknowledged that HIV was extensively present among a wide cross section of American youth. Officials and the public expressed alarm, but instead of revising their conviction that real citizens need not heed Surgeon Generals' warnings, the CDC proclaimed its intention to "target youth," accelerating the nascent effort to carve up America's youth into groups to which different lessons would be taught. Despite the fleeting moment when Magic Johnson talked tough on the Arsenio Hall Show in November of 1991, the damage had already been done. The national pedagogy consolidated the path to citizenship as one that skirted the dangerous zone of HIV infection and opposed compassion with the possibility of infection.

As one compassionate citizen pedagogue would advise other parents:

For teenagers, then, there must be two types of AIDS education. One provides young people with the factual information regarding the nature of the disease, its means of transmission, and the precautions one should take to avoid contracting it. The second type deals with the attitudes teenagers should adopt toward people with AIDS. (Elkind 1990: 192)

In reality, the first kind of education had been made virtually impossible by the restrictions that prevented discussion of condoms or instruction in nonintercourse forms of sex. The right wing's demand to "teach" abstinence created the next generation's paradox: equating "no sex" and safe sex suggests that no sex is safe.

2

Between Innocence
and Safety

Although only a small proportion of teenagers are at high risk for contracting AIDS, a
majority — like my sons — will probably have at least passing acquaintance with a
person who contracts or dies from the disease.

David Elkind, "What Teens Know about AIDS"

Paradoxically, the national pedagogy that provided an identity for adult citizens delayed the identification of their children as potentially at risk. By the
time AIDS education and especially safe sex education in the schools became
topics of national debate, nearly 250,000 young people had contracted HIV.
But their peers — the people from whom they might draw support and with
whom they might have sex and share their intimate lives — were still largely
deprived of desperately needed risk reduction advice.

By 1990, 6,233 cases of AIDS were reported in persons aged 20–25, with
an additional 19,568 cases reported in people aged 25–29 (Athey 1991: 523).
Studies of the prevalence of HIV antibody in Army and Job Corps recruits
conducted through the late 1980s showed rates of 0.15 percent nationally,
with rates of 1.6 percent among minority youth in some major cities; studies
among runaway youth in metropolitan areas show rates as high as 10 percent
(Boyer and Kegeles 1991: 12). Since scientists put the average time from
infection to diagnosable symptoms at ten years, the bulk of the 25,701 young
men and women diagnosed with AIDS by 1990 had been infected as teenagers.

Presumably, young people continued to become infected, thus, some larger number were infected but did not present symptoms that would have brought them to the attention of epidemiologists.[1] These scattered data suggest that somewhere between 110,000 and 260,000 Americans in their teens and early twenties were infected with HIV during the first decade of the epidemic.

During this time some attention was devoted to instilling future citizens with a sense of tolerance toward people living with AIDS. But in those crucial first years, when millions of young people were initiating sex and drug use, there was little effort to provide the tools they needed to evaluate and reduce their *own* risk of contracting HIV. There was little encouragement and help for those who were already infected: they knew next to nothing about how to stall the onset of symptoms. The tragic smugness of Dr. Elkind's perception rests on his certainty that "my sons" will not have sex with other men, take up drug injection, or, more generally, have anything but a "passing acquaintance" with people who are living with HIV.

In fact, paternal predictions had a grain of truth, but only because there were already so many subtle forms of sexual ghettoization that served, at least for a time, to isolate a range of "deviant" communities within the larger, class-stratified urban areas. If middle-class suburban straight kids (Ali Geertz was the exception that underscored the rule) were not yet contracting HIV in large numbers, it was only because they, like their parents, did not have sex across race or class lines and found it difficult to construct a homosexual life unless they left home to become the infamous "runaways." Lesbian, gay, and bisexual youth of all classes and colors, and young people bold enough to pursue their desire across class and race boundaries, met in a terra incognita, a social-sexual space with inarticulate mores that probably rarely presumed safe sex. But instead of recognizing its own children among the actors in the sexual brave new world, the white middle class reclassified them as "deviant," as noncitizens: the white middle class sacrificed its own children in order to sustain the collective delusion that citizens must learn compassion but *cannot* contract HIV. Indicting "deviant" individuals, instead of acknowledging the systems of racial and sexual apartheid that generally militate against cross-race and cross-class relations, insulated middle-class white kids more from their social responsibility than from HIV.

From 1985 to 1990, the popular media and, less explicitly, public health information assigned young people to three categories related to their potential for incorporation into the body politic. While the media sometimes used the terms "teenager," "adolescent," and "young adult" interchangeably, each usually had a particular connotation that was tacitly underwritten by the two most common views of adolescence: the raging hormones (or storm and stress) theory and the youth as subculture theory. Each had different notions of the young person's relation to knowledge about "adult" matters, but both assumed the existence of a stage between a natural and innocent childhood and an accomplished, knowing adulthood.

Dominant class youth were described as the "adolescents" of storm and stress theory, while gay teenagers were treated as a subculture anxiously linked both to heterosexual peers and to adult homosexuals. Young people of color were treated through contextual rhetorics that suggested a natural relation between the environment of the ghetto and the black body. Understood as premodern and, therefore, outside either model of adolescence, youth of color were outside the discourse of innocence that veiled and protected their white, heterosexual age-peers. Youth of color neither were subjects who evoked the protective concerns that innocence mobilized nor were they considered capable of participating as full "adults," *as citizens,* in "modern" society.

Initial descriptions of who was at risk of personal dereliction and, thus, infection put "children" out of bounds because of their innocence. Once they headed toward a sexuality, they were presumed heterosexual and simply mapped into the category of those who need not panic.

Beginning in 1985 there was a steady trickle of articles about young people's risk for contracting HIV, which accelerated as the Global Program on AIDS focused its 1989 World AIDS Day (December 1) on youth, commissioning a million dollar film for use around the world. But the pre-1990 shriek and hush cycles about the risk of HIV infection among teens were so confused about whom they meant to address that few young people recognized themselves as the targets of risk reduction messages. Educators had a hard time figuring out how to address young people without igniting sexual desires that, adults believed, might otherwise have lain safely fallow: they did not know if they could extend the mantle of safety that heterosexuality promised without producing a premature sexuality that might so easily go queer. The incapacity to craft advice was not merely individual adults' discomfort with the topic of

Between Innocence and Safety

sexuality, but government policy, as described by Dr. James Mason, Assistant Secretary of Health and Human Services: "There is no way that the federal government can condone [condom-distribution programs]. It supersedes parental rights, and it sends a direct message to youth that having sex is OK when all our evidence is showing that it isn't. We have to take responsibility for adolescent AIDS" (Brownworth 1992: 44).

Mason's form of government responsibility meant that in the national public, only parents had a right to information about risk reduction: but as compassionate citizens, they had already learned that people like themselves need not worry about contracting HIV. Mason has no interest in the youth who fell outside this protective bubble within the national public: youth who lead sex lives hidden from their parents, and those who had completely departed for the subculture of homosexuals or sex workers. Tragically, for many youths who might eagerly have taken nonjudgmental and straightforward information under advisement, adult equivocation proved homocidal. The national obsession with sexual deviance (whether in the form of homosexuality or of "premature" sex) produced the HIV epidemic among youth by promoting horror at youth sexuality rather than calm advice to young people. Instead of avidly and voyeuristically describing "children's" sexual practices in order to provide detailed prevention advice, as they had done when "scientifically" studying HIV among gay men and prostitutes, the government and media averted their eyes from the fact of young people's sexual practice. Instead, epidemiologists and government policymakers focused their attention on enumerating the routes of transmission (sex, drugs, blood products) of those young people already infected. They counted dying bodies instead of recognizing the reason why young people became infected. The national pedagogy had provided no clear, applicable risk reduction information to youth; the growing cult of Christian family values and the schools that acquiesced to it impeded the formation of local, collective — even dissident — norms of safe sex.

The "safe" alternatives offered to youth — abstinence, condoms, or "mutual masturbation" (now a virtual perversion) — were overdetermined choices when opposed to the newly articulated practice now prescribed for the citizen: adult, latex-free, penile-vaginal intercourse with someone who had been chosen carefully — ordinary sex with ordinary people. Unless the individual had never had sex, abstinence hinged safety on the assurance of serostatus and promoted obsessive testing instead of calm mastery of transmission-interrupting techniques. Condoms were difficult for young people to obtain: they had to choose between safe sex and parental wrath. Multiplying by two (God forbid imagining orgies of multiple masturbation) the denigrating and stop-gap practice of "getting off" alone, "mutual masturbation," a cluster of activities engaged in by adults for a wide range of reasons (from dislike of intercourse to temporary deviations of aim caused by menstruation, male impotence, injury, or boredom), seemed inhumanly sterile instead of blissfully fluid-free. Having valorized penile-vaginal intercourse as the sine qua non of transcendent body-fusion, the elusive and never explained "mutual masturbation" seemed second-rate to young people responding to the lure of emotional intimacy and, perhaps, of orgasms with each other.

This value-laden framing of safe sex had consequences. Studies published as early as 1988 clearly showed that young people were knowledgeable about routes of transmission, but still lacked information about prevention. Studies continue to show that young people are confused about the value of condoms in preventing HIV transmission. A cluster of Boston-based studies of teens' behaviors and perceptions were fairly typical of this form of research, though the findings may not be as bleak as other major cities, given that Boston public health agencies and inner-city service and community groups have been unusually active in preventing STDs, teen pregnancy, drug use, and, by the late 1980s, HIV, through media campaigns and peer education projects. A Commonwealth of Massachusetts Department of Public Health study (CMDPH 1990) found the statewide average age of first intercourse to be sixteen years, with a somewhat younger average in the urban centers. Thirty-two percent of the sexually active teens reported sometimes using condoms, while 37 percent reported never using condoms, with 20 percent of this latter group having unprotected intercourse with multiple partners.

Statewide STD rates among teens had doubled since 1985; Boston teens have gonorrhea infection rates nearly seven times higher than the state average for all ages. In addition, 1 percent of Bostonians between the ages of ten and twenty-four had chlamydia, 17 percent of inner-city births were to teen mothers, and an estimated 10 percent of the Commonwealth's teenage females became pregnant annually. Although HIV seroprevalence studies specifically of adolescents had not been undertaken, back calculation of diagnosed AIDS cases and data from army recruits suggested that seroprevalence rates among Boston teens were somewhere between one-tenth and three-tenths of 1 percent in 1990 (DHH 1992), with out-of-school and homeless youth thought to engage in higher rates of risk activity and thus believed to have higher rates of HIV seroprevalence. An anecdotal report from an agency serving these youth said that about 10 percent of their clients had revealed that they knew they were HIV seropositive (Boston AIDS Consortium 1991).

Drug use by adolescents has not been as well documented; however, the CMDPH (1990) study showed that approximately 3 to 4 percent of Boston teens initiated drug injection annually, and more than half of those who had ever injected a drug shared their needles. Since injection requires a certain amount of expertise, those initiating injection commonly rely on longer-term users to "hit" them, a period of apprenticeship and dependence that can last for months or years, especially in the case of female injectors who are dependent on males (Rosenbaum and Murphy 1990). Due to historical patterns of drug traffic, young inner-city males are at highest risk for beginning injection drug use and for involving peers in injection drug use. Drug use and needle sharing represent important social bonds and tests of group membership among young men, and to a lesser but growing degree, their female friends and partners (Battjes and Pickens 1988; Ramos 1990).

Although American teens score high on tests of the basic information that has been available in "the general public," few perceive themselves to be at risk. Some do not understand the efficacy of particular risk reduction techniques, and many rely on vague partner selection strategies or simply believe that for themselves infection will be a matter of luck. Statewide surveys (Hingson et al. 1990; DHH 1992) show that among Boston youth about half believed that they could not contract HIV through any form of sex with someone who "looks healthy," about a third did not know that abstinence from sex reduced risk of transmission, and 15 percent did not know that condoms reduce HIV transmission.

Multiply these fatal gaps in knowledge and clearly established patterns of behaviors that are HIV transmission enabling by the some 56,000 teenagers in Boston, and there was solid evidence of a clear and present problem. Given that teens as a normative group continually gain new members, and given that most teens initiate sex, and to a lesser extent, drug use with peers, Boston, and cities like it, had clearly documented the makings of an ongoing public health disaster. Yet, despite the increasingly bleak pictures of youth networks as potential sites for rapid dispersion of HIV, public health officials were slow to define young people as a group for intensified and innovative education.

One reason why concern about young people was slow to emerge had to do with the evolution of scientific understanding about a syndrome that was so early and firmly associated with adults and adult sexuality. It was not until the mid-1980s, following the discovery of HIV and review of epidemiologic data — especially the stored serum from a cohort of thousands of gay men who had been enrolled in a hepatitis B study begun in 1978 — that researchers were able to realize that time from infection to AIDS diagnosis might be a decade or more. Only then was it indisputable that people diagnosed in their early to mid-twenties must have been infected as teenagers. However, the media's framing of early concerns about young people suggest that additional cultural factors prevented the constitution of teens *as a class* of people at special risk of contracting HIV through sex.

The initial articles addressing young people and HIV infection took two forms. The first were reports about whether infected "school children" should be allowed in the classroom (*Time* 1985a, 1985b, 1986). Represented as having been infected through transfusions or from blood products used in conjunction with clotting disorders, teenagers were lumped together with elementary school children because their route of transmission was considered the same: nonsexual, iatrogenic, *innocent.*

The most tenured figure in the school debates was Ryan White, whose life with HIV was widely documented in the popular press. White initially came to the nation's attention at age thirteen when he was banned from school and hooked up to his classrooms via telephone. We watched White grow into early manhood, which included getting a girlfriend and becoming friends with rock stars like Michael Jackson and Elton John. While there were occasional comments in interviews that he was being sexually cautious with his girlfriend, White, like men with clotting disorders generally, was never represented as a sexual being. His passage through adolescence seemed to keep him in a state of perpetual innocence: the terror of sexually active HIV-infected teenagers never emerged.

The second area of coverage of teens and HIV concerned whether or not college students were "practicing safe sex" (*Newsweek* 1985; van Gelder and Brandt 1986). While representations of their suspect decision-making practices abounded, the fact of their sexual activity loomed larger than the issue of

Between Innocence and Safety

their youthfulness. At least initially, the *age* of students seemed less a concern than their potential promiscuity: college students were treated within the larger concern about "heterosexual AIDS" in the wake of Rock Hudson's death.

In all of these cases, concerns centered on white, working/middle-class young people, most of whom were "straight." Occasionally, articles included an account of a now infected gay-boy-next-door. But these accounts were less worried about his possible cross-age, same-sex sexuality than they were intent on describing a clueless middle America that had no language to talk about sex, much less any interest in ensuring that its children were "safe." Both *Rolling Stone* (van Gelder and Brandt 1986) and the *New York Times* (Gross 1987) produced rare articles that went into detail about the views and situation of young gay men. But by desexualizing the youth, each article partially rescues "gay teen-agers, . . . many of them are not yet sexually active" (Gross 1987: B1) from the category "deviant" by considering them a subcategory of *students,* "gay men of college age" (van Gelder and Brandt 1986), that is, a hidden part of the citizenry-in-the-making.

If stories that allowed nice gay boys to be counted as the nation's innocent teens suggested that homophobia had diminished, racism and sexism quickly filled the vacated space. Epidemiologic data clearly showed that among men of color reported as having AIDS, a large percentage must have contracted HIV in their teens. Likewise, a significant percentage of women generally, but especially women of color, diagnosed with AIDS must have contracted HIV as teens. However, young people of color were never represented as part of the nation's future citizens, despite the fact that they were the very group whose bodies would be a critical force in the Gulf War. Not only were they not counted as "teens" or "students," they were excluded from the discourse of innocence that defined which lives might be worth saving. Instead, youth of color, like the adults into whom they would imperceptibly merge, were colonized through metaphors that equated the U.S. ghetto with an Africa now ravaged by AIDS.

Even in this early coverage, the connotative meanings associated with terms for the young began to divide into the same rough categories that had emerged to describe who was at risk among adults. The adolescent of AIDS discourse was the "normally abnormal," hormone-besieged body of the white working/middle-class youth. The "at risk" teen was either gay or a member of the black/latin urban underclass and was presumably involved in drugs and prostitution. Understood as autonomous groups of young people, the "at risk" teens were represented as a source of danger and not a site of innocence.

This discourse of innocence, sexuality, and HIV risk would not become fully legible as an issue of age until the early 1990s. Pediatric cases were analyzed and studied separately but were not considered a true "risk group" because, since most had been infected perinatally, the target of risk reduction education was their mothers. In the case of school attenders, while the possibility of casual transmission was considered an age-related issue (innocent of themselves as "dangerous," young children might drool on or bite other children), and sexual maturity was in question with experimenting college students, the actual grouping together of similarly aged people into the cross-transmission route risk category "adolescent" did not occur until the early 1990s. The idea that youth were at risk intensified with Magic Johnson's November 1991 announcement that he was HIV positive.

The basic logic for separating the young deviant from the "normally abnormal" adolescent, and thereby determining who needs to know about safe sex, depended on the construction of normal adolescence as a passage from a precultural body (the innocent child), through a civilizing process (the adolescent with desires but without practices), to a sexually responsible adulthood (heterosexual, monogamous, married, procreative, white). The media constituted two deviations from this developmental tale: black bodies never passed through culture, having neither adolescence nor civilized adulthood; similarly, homosexual bodies passed through adolescence, but emerged into a distinct subculture associated with foreclosed adulthood. For both, once deviant sexual practice had occurred, the body could no longer be entered into the national public except as object of scrutiny or compassion.

"Normally Abnormal"

Anna Freud described the period between childhood and adulthood as a time of upheaval and liminality in which the normal and abnormal are reversed: "To be normal during the adolescent period is by itself abnormal" (1958:

275). Even critics of the older versions of this theory view "the study of adolescence [as] fundamentally the study of change" (Powers, Hauser, and Kilner 1989: 202). In its many guises and revisions, this broad paradigm grounds human development in bio-psychological terms whose rhetorical force lies in the analogy presumed between the biological process of literal and linear "growth" and the psychological process of "development." These are in turn analogized to the "progress" of civilization itself. This conflation of starkly biological, psychological, and cultural change shows modernist thought at its most compressed, simultaneously an epistemology and a hermeneutic. The narrative tropes of development, the beginning and the ending, constitute a binary opposition joined through a transitional middle. This tripartite structure is not a dialectic in any usual sense: far from constituting the uplifting, canceling-while-preserving synthesis of Hegelian *Aufhebung,* the phase that joins the innocence of childhood/prerationality/primitive with adulthood/rationality/civilization is a crisis phase embodying the *worst* of both worlds. As manifested in storm and stress theory, the teleogical overdrive of the three phases scrambles the middle figure in order to produce the originary "past" as unknowable to the adult: the semblance of dialectical tension between childhood innocence and the wisdom of age helps underwrite the power adults have over the interpretation of the now-impossible-to-remember experience of the body before sexuality. The metaphors made available by the developmental narrative valorize adult/mature/civilized knowledge claims over their Other: psychological subjectivity, moral reasoning, and political agency are conveyed only to those at the outer reaches of the teleological parade, tautologically figured as and explained as proper to the "big."

When mapped onto the body, storm and stress theory argues that the physiological changes occurring in the adolescent body are in danger of outstripping the young person's reasoning capacities. Sexuality, properly but precariously comprised of innocent pleasure and adult responsibility, becomes a source of tremendous anxiety for society and individual. The most viscerally appealing image of the physiological crisis of adolescent sexuality is contained, of course, in the reportage about child sexual abuse. The crime of reversing or transgressing the teleology of sexual maturation is figured as adult-sized penises penetrating the as-yet-too-small orifices of the ungendered child (it seems not to matter much whether the space in danger of violent penetration is a mouth, vagina, or anus).

Sigmund Freud compellingly argued that childhood is marked by forms of desire that ought to count as sexuality, indeed, these unself-conscious somatic pleasures *are* innocence. By contrast, America of the 1980s, crowned by the national AIDS pedagogy, insisted that *real* sex — intercourse — requires a self-reflexive recognition that this *is* (the potentially dangerous) sex. Contrary to the folklore that having intercourse conveys, at least, manhood, HIV education for adolescents argued that it is not the act of sex itself that produces adult status, but having sex when you are old enough to know what you are doing. The often invoked female-bodies-too-small-for-childbearing — "babies having babies" — stand for bodies driven by pleasures that they lack the moral capacity to manage. Even when represented as "big enough," girls' own bodies ("early physical development," according to an advice column to be examined later) put them at risk by attracting the attention of the "big" penises that simultaneously take pleasure and convey "consequences" for which the girl-child cannot be prepared — carnal knowledge, pregnancy, and now, HIV-infection.

A typical pamphlet *about* (but not directed *to*) adolescents, produced by Burroughs-Wellcome,[2] cites (in a footnote to the term "moral reasoning") the developmental theories of Erik Erickson to warn counselors that

Several factors make counseling of adolescents, especially early adolescents, unusually complicated. People in their early teens tend to have a low level of comfort and familiarity with their bodies, a poor capability to plan for future events and their consequences, and are unable to consider the viewpoints of others. Thus, they are prone to greater risk-taking and are therefore vulnerable to the consequences of their behavior. The development of "moral reasoning" occurs during adolescence. (Burroughs-Wellcome 1989: 17–18)

For adolescents, desire and practice are radically split: they are presumed to only engage in "risk behaviors" if they chance to discover such behaviors exist. They may be naturally subject to changing desires, but these desires are acorporeal and insufficient in themselves to result in sexual behavior. As we will see later in a more extensive discussion of Gina Kolata's (1990) account, adolescents are "thinking about SATs and college," and wouldn't engage in sex unless they were subjected to "pressure" by older people, possibly strangers: "Feeling pressured to fit in with an older crowd, [David Kamens] had unprotected sex with people he did not know well" (149). But these "adult" pressures may also come from peers, according to Carnegie Council on Adolescent Development policy advocates Jackson and Hornbeck (1989). As innocent bodies en route to differentiation from their parents, some adolescents mimic adult behavior. The danger of adolescence is that "although increased identification with peers serves to fulfill needs for autonomy from parents, it also provides increased pressure to engage in adult behavior such as sex, smoking, and drinking" (833). Falling just short of accusing teens of pressuring each other into untimely pleasures (their identification with each other is separable from the desire to "engage in adult behavior"), the policy analysts repeat the logic of "fitting" across power/knowledge differences described more baldly by Kolata. "Pressure" is applied on the fault line between the quest for autonomy through shared disidentification with parents and the group performance of the very behaviors that mark their parents as adults. This is the logic of psychosexual development: some magic threshold must be collectively crossed before young people can safely engage in the pursuit of pleasure together.

Virtually everyone agrees that adolescents should be educated "about AIDS" before they fall prey to their hormones and to the complex negotiation of adult status glossed as "rebelliousness" on its way to "manhood." Unlike black or gay youth, whose representations I will describe in a moment, the national pedagogy imagined that white heterosexual youth could be *fully* prevented from starting on the slippery slope to risk behaviors if only they can be prevented from "experimenting." Adolescents must learn about heterosexual practice *just after* they land securely within the heterosexual mainstream. If they "learn about AIDS" they will not need know about (much less practice) safe sex: being the subject who must learn about AIDS (rather than about safe sex) enters the adolescent body into the category of future citizen (as opposed to a future "social problem"). Knowing about or practicing safe sex *produces* danger, is symptomatic of the perversion or the premature heterosexuality that is certain to derail the adolescent body from its quest for citizenship.

The national pedagogy set itself a difficult task: preserve the central category of mainstream or public as naturally and literally HIV-free and provide a conduit for youth to enter it HIV-free, but without practicing safe sex. The mute strategy was to keep adolescents away from "bad influences" who might prematurely introduce the idea of sex, thus providing a concrete outlet for their raging hormones that would result in exposure to HIV. But if sexual contact with others was too scary, might not these HIV-free heterosexuals acquire a species-destroying fear of sex, even with the right people?[3] Sustaining the idea that latex-free intercourse was the reward for the patriot, while "safe sex" was a punishment for any number of deviants, required a series of strange lessons about the biomechanics of HIV transmission. The image of perverts transgressing cultural borders was superimposed on descriptions of the biology of mucous membranes and viral particles. Virus-membrane contact became a metaphor for sexual invasion across the cordon sanitaire between the public and subcultures. Biology was less real than sociology: seeing supposed deviants was equated with taking infected fluids into the most private recesses of one's body. As Elkind's description hints, being compassionate toward people usually despised is a small price to pay to avoid the humiliation and dehumanization of safe sex.

Like the ancillary lectures on which students will never be quizzed, these lessons began by introducing the idea of safe sex (now reduced to the disgusting, condom-ridden acts of perverts), only to reassure white teens that they need not have more than an abstract knowledge of it as long as they maintained the requirements of citizenship that would shield them from real risk. The emphasis on the improbability of contracting HIV through casual contact and the calls to civility toward people living with AIDS, coupled with the lack of clear information on prevention (especially condom use), positioned the adolescent consumer of AIDS education as someone who *can't* be infected. Any lingering anxiety about their proximity to deviants — "social contact" — is offset: compassion erases the panic that one might discover a hidden desire to have sex *with* them. Intrinsic to the notion of civility toward people living with AIDS was the idea that they are *different* — not white, not straight, not anyone toward whom the adolescent would experience sexual desire.

By 1990, the heterosexual, white working/middle-class adolescent was both the target of and defined by education that emphasized abstinence and advocated the development of personal systems for weeding out risky partners. Hot on the heels of twenty-three-year-old Ali Geertz's announcement that she had contracted HIV from a "nice" boy of her same (upper middle) class, Kolata (1990) argued that the mistaken association of HIV infection with deviance — even with deviant teenagers — had misled *Seventeen* magazine's readers (largely teenage girls): "A year and a half ago more than half the teenagers Dr. Hein saw at her clinic were street kids who had run away from home or had been kicked out and who often were prostitutes, having sex with many partners and injecting drugs. Now more than half the teenagers she sees are living at home with their families or are college students" (150).

But the unspoken strategy of keeping "nice" kids away from bad influences was hard to shake. The article also included the story of infected teenager turned safe sex educator W. David Kamens, a "nice boy" who went to dance school. He embodies the teen whose physical precociousness resulted in joining an "older crowd" who pressure him to do "adult" things for which he was emotionally unequipped:

Other teenagers think that if they know the person they're having sex with, they don't have to worry about AIDS. But your sex partner may not tell you about all of his previous sexual experiences. David Kamens . . . started hanging around with an older crowd and didn't ask much about his new friends' sexual experiences. . . . "I really didn't know what I was doing." (151)

Kamens operates both as the positive figure of the unsuspecting teen and, although the gender of his sexual partners is unstated, as the negative figure of danger. We don't know if he is describing himself or the partner who infected him when he says: "You really can't tell whether a boy is infected with HIV by looking at him or even talking to him" (151). Other journalists treat Kamens, whose AIDS education efforts afforded him a brief national profile, as a member of a subculture, the more common construction of gay teenagers. For example, Brownworth (1992) describes him as openly gay and actively involved in advocating for gay teenagers.

By the late 1980s, the generalized adolescent had emerged as a bodiless vessel of troubling desires whose cognitive capacities were not sufficient to allow for safe decisions. Until they crossed over into full adulthood, their best option was categorical avoidance of older and deviant people. By inscribing and being inscribed by their need to have knowledge of safe sex, two deviant bodies, one homosexual and one black (or "Hispanic"), constituted the visible boundaries of the dimly etched container of the "normal" adolescent. Gay teens, as we will see in the next section, made deviance visible through the notion of subculture. Black and Hispanic youth defined the mainstream through geography and time — through being elsewhere and premodern.

Youth as Subculture

A second important concept of youth emerged in relation to both mid-twentieth-century anthropological investigations of adolescence in other cultures (Mead 1935; Turner 1967) and the popular post–World War II image of the "rebel without a cause." By the time of the 1960s student movements, it was easy to press the claim that young people were not merely bodies driven by hormones, but a class, an inexplicable *culture* on the other side of a "generation gap." Mead's comparative work showed that "stress" is not a universal feature of "adolescence" but a cultural construct with widely variable meanings. Turner's work of the 1960s analyzed the symbols and practices of child-to-adult transformation among Ndembu, who, he argued, saw the transition less as a bio-psychological developmental phase than a temporary and separate state of being. Turner's "liminal phase" suggested that the very idea of bio-psychological process might be a cultural construct, a displacement into the individual's body of the *social* transformation of "children" into "adults." The influence of these two works extended far beyond the academy: Mead was widely read and extremely popular among lay readers, and Turner, though perhaps less widely read by the public, was something of a cult figure among young intellectuals in the academic boom years of the late-sixties to mid-seventies.

These trends in popular intellectual circles neatly converged with a more general shift in post–World War II society. The new category of teen mediated the huge economic shifts that occurred when veterans — "teens" of the previous generation — displaced the women and black men who had migrated to cities to work in factories during the war effort. Women were redomesticated through the invention of a largely white suburban lifestyle, while unemployed blacks increasingly populated the inner cities. Teen culture created a new consumption center, while eliminating suburban youth from the job market. Post-World War II anxiety and nostalgia helped establish the new category of teenager. Rebellious white boys ("Rebel[s] without a Cause") were both a threat to small town life as it had been ("The Wild Ones") but also an extension of the frontiersman to the modern world. Their black age-peers were simply considered men without jobs. Technological advances in leisure activity, and the emerging emphasis on consumption, meant that by the 1950s, products were developed and marketed directly to "teens," especially to those in the white middle class. Although they did not benefit financially, un- or underemployed black age-peers became a primary source of the new white youth culture of rock and roll.

Youth began to be viewed as a social role, less importantly tied to physiology than to the economic and social mandates that governed entry into adult social roles. The teenager was associated with "modern" society and "modern attitudes"; they consumed new cultural products like rock and roll and automobiles, and rebelled against prevailing norms of sexual and substance-use austerity. Youth were tacitly understood as a subculture, defined by their attitudes and patterns of consumption. Sexuality was still a principal concern with teens, but youth culture began to assert a discourse of its own. Sexuality was dangerous not because there was a mind (morality)/body (hormonal) mismatch, but because of the sexual *neuroses* that arose from the perceived repressiveness of the 1950s: puritanical adult society was the source of sexual danger. To youth liberationists[4] and a fascinated popular media, the sexual body had to be protected, not from the unreasoning adolescent mind, but from the moralizing attitudes of an adult culture that hated, instead of celebrated, the "natural" (i.e., sexual, pleasurable) body. Despite its emphasis on young people's own values, the idea of subcultures only partially challenged the teleology of storm and stress theory: 1960s youth activism politicized the sexual body and shifted the power to control it toward youth, but only temporarily. The youth liberation movement dwindled by the 1970s (to be partially revived in the 1980s by gay/lesbian/bisexual youth activism and by the political wing of rap musicians) because the adult-youth dichotomy it retained had an inherent time limitation. Activists who were now adults could no longer press their claims to self-determination on a new generation of oppressed youth who seemed intent on copying the conservative mores liberationists had once opposed.

Theories that see youth as a subculture often also see youth culture as a space of resistance, as in the work of mid-1970s Birmingham Center scholars like Dick Hebdige (1979) and Angela McRobbie (1991). The widely distributed English version of the Danish youth movement's *The Little Red Schoolbook* (Roberts 1971) is a classic example of youth liberation rhetoric:

This is an Americanized version of a British translation of a Danish book. That it was possible to take a book written about the schools of one nation and that had been rewritten and translated to describe the schools of a second nation and use it to describe the schools of a third nation, without either distorting reality or changing the content or tone of the book substantially, illustrates an important and disturbing fact about schools in Europe and North America: they are basically the same, and the sameness is a poor quality education and an unjust educational system.

The purpose of the book is to provide you with some basic information that will help you deal with that fact . . . [and] to provide you with information which you can't usually get in school or from most grown-ups — about sex and drugs, for instance — and to give you some ideas about how you can use the schools for your purposes so that you can really have what schools have always promised the young but hardly ever delivered: power over their own lives. (15–16)

Here, youth, or those who have just recently been youth, offer information — "about sex and drugs, for instance" — which is described as having been monitored by adults and their institutions in order to control youth. In this framework, *giving information* is intrinsically empowering and political because it leads to young people taking "power over their own lives." Significantly, while the youth movement has declined in number, or at least visibility, adults who provide services *to* youth continue in this ethos, which they may have experienced in their own youth. For example, youth advocate Gabe Kruks, director of public policy and planning for the Gay and Lesbian Community Services Center of Los Angeles, is among those who place the major blame for youth's plight on society, not on hormones:

We really have to start looking at kids' needs instead of our own. We have the highest rate of teenage pregnancy, teenage STDs, teenage AIDS, and teenage date rape in the Western world here in the US. We are, as a society, uncomfortable with our bodies, with sex, with sexuality. We're in denial about a lot of issues associated with these subjects. We like to pretend they don't exist. That denial is killing our kids. The US is a very child-hating society. If we were not aware of that before, we can see it very clearly in our response to AIDS. (Brownworth 1992: 43)

Between Innocence and Safety

51

However, while challenging the "normally abnormal" definition used in psycho-physiologically based theories of adolescence, youth-as-subculture theory still views these years as a liminal phase during which young people attempt to acquire the knowledge necessary to becoming adults. Subculture theorists believe that adult culture tries to prevent youth from learning what they need to know (especially about sex), and, thus, youth culture needs to be nourished so that youth can share "accurate" and "appropriate" knowledge among themselves. This creates a paradox for radical youth advocates. On one hand, they are trying to protect youth from an adult culture of which they are members. But on the other hand, they feel the need to ensure that youth knowledge is "accurate," requiring adults' active involvement in the youth community and its self-protective languages and mores. Replacing the temporary insanity model with a Marxian false consciousness model adds a veneer of progressive politics, but this ineluctable generational power relation leaves the adult in the position of interpreting the youth's development toward a state in which he (and for youth advocates, *she*) can make good decisions about sexuality.

Representations of youth that come from this perspective have to work around the fact of adults' greater control over image production. Brownsworth's "Teen Sex: America's Worst-Kept Secret" (1992), which appeared in a major national gay news magazine, places the subculturalist politic in the mouths of youth who seem to state its terms naturally. Using profiles of teens living with AIDS, Brownworth indicts families rather than peers, reinforcing youth's solidarity in the face of a hostile adult society. For example, the "perfect California Girl, infected with HIV at age 16," describes her family as "almost too strict about sex" and says "the kid I got this from didn't know any more than I did" (44). A storm and stress theorist could only have interpreted these statements as fearful evidence of young people's incapacity to recognize the misadjustment between their bodies and their moral capacities. But Brownworth's "Perfect California Girl" offers this implicit rebuttal: "Kids aren't embarrassed to have sex, so we should stop making them embarrassed to have safe sex. I want the words *sex* and *condoms* to go together like cereal and milk or peanut butter and jelly" (44).

By the late 1980s, the mainstream media used the subculture notion almost exclusively in reference to gay youth. Despite numerous contemporaneous articles about mainstream youth's fashions, musical preferences, or sheer inexplicability, when it came to AIDS reportage, the media seemed anxious to distance (adult?) readers from risk, avoiding the possibility that heterosexual youth were part of a (the same?) subculture. These mainstream accounts inverted the radical advocates' concept to argue that some youth were at risk *because* they belonged to a subculture. Heterosexual youth were by definition outside subculture, now overdetermined by its sexual rather than its stylistic element. Even Brownworth's *Advocate* article inadvertently split "straight" and "gay" teens into a mainstream and a subculture. Describing a real case of the queer paradigm (Patton 1985a, 1985b), in which queers are presumed to "have AIDS" and in which anyone who contracts HIV is presumed to have engaged in queer acts, Brownworth uncovers the societal incapacity to think outside the categories of "ordinary" and "deviant"; the "perfect California girl," once infected, finds herself incorporated into the subculture of the original queers: "I finally ended up being placed with Gay and Lesbian Adolescent Social Services in L.A. I wasn't gay, but they were the only place that would take me" (44).

"Gay" Teenagers

Breaking from the usual policy (until about 1991) of refusing to use the term "gay," the *New York Times* ran two prominent articles (Gross 1987; Eckholm 1990) on "gay teenagers" that constructed as an autonomous group the young (white) men who were naturally discovering their unnatural sexualities in the age of AIDS. Oddly, the author still refers to adults as "homosexuals": evidently the *Times* wished to evade the sexuality of the "teens" who might have desires and feelings, but must not be spoken of as engaging in sexual practices, despite the fact that key figures in each story had already contracted HIV. The article carefully balances two oppositions — gay-straight, adult-teen — in order to retain the adult homosexual as a dangerous and isolated individual while drawing a protective border around those teens whom the middle class prefers to view as more endangered than dangerous: the boy next door might suffer the tragedy of AIDS but is never imaged to be infectious himself.

The term "gay teen" suggests a self-conscious group bound together by common experience, rather than isolated individuals who merely come together for the purpose of having sex. The young men's special experience of their deviant desires, rather than perverted practices in themselves, seems to form the basis for group identification. Gay teens are

a population in turmoil, bearing all the problems common to adolescence and another set all their own. These gay teen-agers run the gamut from inconspicuous youngsters in high school who are isolated and frightened by their stirring sexuality to runaways on the piers of Greenwich Village who openly sell themselves as prostitutes. (Gross 1987: B1)

Paradoxically, gay teens are granted the "right" to sex, but largely in order to specify *which* teens, even in mainstream America, are subject to AIDS. The gay teenager (who is almost always male) achieves media visibility not for his own benefit, but in order to inscribe the heterosexual teen as safe from AIDS. The homosexuality of gay teens is fixed by describing them as members of a subculture. Removed from both the mainstream heterosexual and from the adult gay "communities," their diverse community, or rather communities, are distinct from mainstream society. Whatever they do, gay teens' present or future practices are rendered as separate from the activity of their heterosexual peers; the line between gay and non-gay youth is irrevocable: "Experts agree that the fear of AIDS will not convert a gay youngster to heterosexuality, but they might slow a decision to have intercourse" (B1).

The *Times* concedes an almost natural category of gay teens but implicitly suggests that the specter of HIV infection for such young men lies in liaison with adults and not in "experiments" among themselves. This fatal perception, which duplicates the "little hole" logic in queer terms, is held by gay (and straight) teens and underwrites the media cannibalizing of Eddie Savitz discussed in the next chapter. This logic promotes subculturalist understanding among youth, even while adults see them through the raging hormone lens. The *Times* reinforces youth's mistaken belief in the safety of their peers, while playing on updated stereotypes about ruthless older men who pursue young men. Youth are encouraged to view their friends as nonrisky, while adults are encouraged to view their aura of innocence as the source of their potential victimization by older men or "precocious" peers. The coverage relies wholly on the partner selection logic promoted to the national public.

The fatal logic that HIV is more common in older people serves two roles: to justify not explaining the mechanics of safe sex to young people, and to open up the specter of pedophilic monsters who are following the fatal advice and carefully choosing young people who lack sexual history and, presumably, lack HIV.

As we will see in the next chapter, the danger of pedophilia in the 1980s is not simply that pedophiles are seeking out youth, but that they are now searching for lower risk rather than simple innocence. Despite the fact that they were enacting the very logic of safe sex promoted by the national pedagogy, these men, presumed infected (but how, if they only have sex with youth?), are now seen as the very worst sort of pervert:

Many [gay teens] are not yet sexually active, but others wind up in physical relationships they are not prepared for. . . . Social workers say the men who buy [gay teens'] favors, and sometimes carry infection home to their wives, are seeking progressively younger partners in the hope they will be "clean." (Gross 1987: B1)

Equivocating on who infects whom, this *Times* writer is, in comparison with other articles about bisexual men, suddenly concerned about the young men whom it otherwise vilifies as the *source* of infections to the unknowing wives of the men who purchase their services. Despite the admission that "huge numbers [of adult homosexuals] have adopted 'safer sex' " (Eckholm 1990: A1), the *Times* neatly ignores the possibility that young men might as easily learn *about* safe sex from their encounters with older men, peer education at its most basic. Apparently, noncommercial relations with homosexual partners who practice safe sex are *more* risky to gay youth than are commercial transactions with bisexual johns who attempt to shield themselves from risk by searching for markers of youth instead of donning condoms.

This construction of the gay teen creates a pedagogic paradox: you can't teach him to be gay, since pedagogy only creates citizens, but you don't want him to become a counterfeit citizen — a bisexual — who serves as the bridge between straight and gay, who introduces HIV into the mainstream through "ordinary" sex. Thus, it is not in school, the usual site of pedagogy, but in the "grim, nether world" in which "smoothfaced youngsters . . . sell themselves for $10" that the most education for gay teens has occurred, even according to the *Times*. The invisible community of the "less troubled" who have

" 'passed' as heterosexual" "have no contact with counselors and receive limited sex education" (Gross 1987). Like their straight peers, the only education these gay teens encounter preaches quixotic personal strategies of avoidance. It is not lost on gay youth that this education is addressed to straight teens about people like themselves; if they learn anything, it is that in the already stigmatized (adult) community for which they are destined, "[AIDS] makes the stakes higher" (Gross 1987).

The right to sex, implied by the growing ease in alluding to gay teens' sexuality, is won only at the cost of making gay youth ultimately responsible for their own fate. No matter how much they evidence a willingness to practice safe sex, gay teens are thought of as prospective homosexual adults who cannot know enough to be safe: "Even young men who are better adjusted and well informed about acquired immune deficiency syndrome may not fully understand that almost any unprotected sex may be suicidal" (Eckholm 1990: B20). Always at risk, but rarely described as infecting anyone else, gay teens exist in a one-way economy of HIV infection: their sex is a gambit of self-destruction. Thus, like their older brothers, for whom devastation is considered a done deed, gay teens are seen as inevitably on the verge of sliding into dangerous practices. Even efforts at salvaging remnants of an alternative pedagogy within gay culture are interpreted by the media as in themselves fatal. A sidebar to *Newsweek*'s 1990 "The Future of Gay America" describes young gays as engaging in a "pro-sex" campaign very reminiscent of the "night life and sexual freedom that defined the disco and bathhouse hedonism of the '70s" (22), which is often implicitly or explicitly situated as the "cause" of AIDS. Apparently because of its affinity to now maligned gay culture, such efforts are destined to fail. In order to dismiss the self-education and grassroots resistance efforts of young queers, the article proposes an "appropriate" gay youth whose conservative style advertises his only hope for safety.

The partial acceptance of white gay youth came at the price of indicting another group of young Americans. Despite equivocation about what a "nice gay boy" might be like, situating him partially within the dominant culture set up youth of color, long rejected from the body politic, as the most vivid example of the "real" problem of AIDS and the young. Social psychology had provided a comfortable framework for explaining away the potentially risky behavior of mainstream heterosexual youth: any danger resulted from the volatile collision of raging hormones and unsavory types, which was abetted by explicit safe sex education. Subculture theory allowed mainstream society to acknowledge gay youth without taking responsibility for educating them. Maintaining distance between the compassionate citizen and the growing HIV-related morbidity and mortality among youth of color required a yet different frame. Both the storm and stress theory and the subcultural theory envisioned their object within civilization. This left a whole range of rhetorics that could describe a premodern, uncivilized human growth process that produced sexual subjects even less able to enter the citizenry.

"Where the Trouble Is": The Premodern Body

Although considered geographically separate from the white mainstream, youth of color presented a more terrifying prospect than the potentially proximate gay youth, the "inconspicious youngsters" (Gross 1987), whose identity as firmly if fatally gay meant that a polymorphous bisexual phase would not transport HIV across the "natural" barrier between the gay and straight worlds. The specter of third-world-like AIDS fueled the new racist paranoia, which situated rampant drug use and random killing — "epidemics" of addiction and violence — as proper to, but threatening to explode out of, the "ghetto." This spatial phantasm operated in tandem with the rhetorical move in Western discourse about AIDS in Africa more generally (Patton 1990, 1992a). Constituting Africa or the ghetto as a displaced geographical space in which "primitive" or "premodern" heterosexual practices are the cause of an irreversible natural disaster legitimated the failure to provide education and to distance, in this case, white heterosexual youth from risk. Their heterosexuality was "ordinary," "civilized." Heterosexual risk lost its specificity — penile-vaginal intercourse — and became equated with premodern sexuality, which is, in Western discourse, a presumptively "black" sexuality. The following description of "the critical transition of adolescence" illustrates the way in which storm and stress theory (and arguably psychoanalytic theories that situate sexual neurosis in relation to "civilization and its discontents") leaves open the possibility of banishing some bodies if they can be counted as premodern:

In premodern times, preparation for adulthood typically extended over much of child-hood. Young people had abundant opportunities for directly observing their parents and other adults performing the adult roles that they would eventually adopt when the changes of puberty endowed them with an adult body and capabilities. The skills necessary for adult life were gradually acquired and fully available, or nearly so, by the end of puberty. (Hamburg and Takanishi 1989: 825)

This apparently innocuous description suggests that in earlier times or other places, the duration or timing of adolescence was not extended forward or backward, but in fact, *never occurred at all.* Childhood, with its early training in adult roles, blended invisibly into adulthood. Virtually everything was learned by the time a now-inconsequential puberty ended. The problem, argue these authors, is that this older system has not been fully supplanted: "In contemporary societies, these social supports have eroded considerably through extensive geographical mobility, scattering of extended families, and the rise of single-parent families, especially those involving very young, very poor, and socially isolated mothers" (825).

The mainstream reader would most certainly associate this and similar invocations of the "broken family" with urban African Americans, already constituted as premodern by virtue of their alleged matriarchal structures, a devastatingly erroneous racist truism scientized with the publication of the 1965 *The Negro Family: The Case for National Action* (collected in Bromley and Longino 1972), more commonly known as the Moynihan report: "In essence, the Negro community has been forced into a matriarchal structure which, because it is so out of line with the rest of the American society, seriously retards the progress of the group as a whole, and imposes a crushing burden on the Negro male and, in consequence, on a great many Negro women as well" (197).

The evocation of families whose children are on a premodern track that circumvents adolescence emerges again in *Psychology Today*'s 1988 cover feature, with its dangerously polysemous title, "The Runaway Epidemic: AIDS on the Streets." Here, the poor family operates as a metonym for the ghetto. The article situates pathology in this family and mobilizes environ-mental rather than cultural metaphors: "Contrary to a lingering perception of runaways as adolescent adventurers, most are victims of dysfunctional families and are fleeing from stressful environments. . . . A picture emerges of deficient youth, lacking the normal states of child growth and development but acting like hardened adults" (Hersch 1988: 31–32). While stories of street youth include descriptions of white youth, the persistent invocation of place and environment — "the extreme danger and stress of street life" (31) — defines the decayed urban core, the supposed domain of communities of color, as the geographically isolated site of a premodern AIDS epidemic. The environment of the ghetto and the urban streets "puts them directly in the path of the disease" (35), making risk apparently unavoidable:

If geography is destiny, runaway and homeless kids gravitate to the very locations around the country where their risk is greatest. Not only are these kids at higher risk with every sexual contact than their suburban counterparts, but they also have higher levels of drug use and sexually transmitted diseases. Often, their immune systems are already compromised by repeated exposure to infections. All of these conditions may increase the risk for developing AIDS. (Hersch 1988: 35)

Like the queer paradigm that assimilated straight kids, the "africanization" inscribed through geographical metaphors includes white street kids. Missing both childhood and adolescence in their premodern trek, street kids and teenagers of color in general are considered "hardened" adults. There is no question of evil outsiders influencing these young people: even if bad parenting is responsible for their diversion from "normally abnormal adolescence," they are now the youth against which the white mainstream is warning their children. Despite its utter pathos, the *Psychology Today* story in part serves to fill in the youthful faces of the category "people to avoid contact with" proposed, but left undefined, in mainstream advice from the Surgeon General's report to family magazines. For example, a *Good Housekeeping* (1990) advice column, in response to the question "Is Your Child at Risk?," provides "markers" as "guides" "to identify youngsters who are at risk." Together with the long-standing psychological problems that might trouble middle-class children — "[G]irls with early physical development" and "[A]dolescents with serious school problems" — the article identifies urban youth as both *at* and a source *of* risk: "Youngsters living in poverty in inner cities are at very high risk. They are often under great social pressures to have sex early, and IV drugs may be rampant in their environment" (257). By collapsing their bodies with the spaces they occupy, young people of color and their africanized white companions are held partially culpable for their fate: they are not *innocent* victims, either because they are said to act like (to "be") adults at much younger ages, or because they live in the harsh inner city, a premodern world in which "primitive" behaviors are expected.

An initially innocent-sounding *New York Times* article that describes a new series of AIDS education films for African American and Hispanic audiences invoked the damning geographic rhetoric in its title, "Putting the AIDS Message Where the Trouble Is" (Yarrow 1989). The article is principally a service feature about the upcoming projects of AIDS Film, whose "AIDS: Changing the Rules" (1987) drew fire from the banana industry because Ruben Blades employed the now-defamed fruit to demonstrate condom use.[5] The writer collapses spectatorial danger with the upcoming films' cultural sensitivity by quoting the company's executive director: he "hoped television broadcasters will be 'bold enough' to show them." The conflict between minority communities' "need to know" and the mainstream's desire not to hear about safe sex serves once again to locate risk in the geographic Other of the ghetto and in the africanized bodies that live there. Implicitly excluded as a potential TV audience for the broadcast, the minority subjects of the film also become a visual Other for the *Times* readers who may tune in to the broadcast.[6] The article goes on to describe black teenagers as living in "a different milieu with different issues." Doubling "different" joins space and problem, reconstituting the mainstream as the "here" and indexing the collection of concerns about being protected *from* as the central problem for the nation and citizen-reader.

Unlike mainstream white adolescents who are to be protected at all costs from frank discussions of sex, youth of color are apparently already possessed by sexual knowledge, whether they have engaged in actual acts or not. Bringing up sex and talking explicitly about drug use is seen as necessary, not culturally insensitive, and certainly not a potential cause of their initiation into sex or drug use. Geographically situated "where the trouble is," the risk faced by youth of color becomes a public, collective phenomenon, rather than a private, individual one. Viewed as hard-to-reach, potentially already lost — "living on the razor's edge with drugs and sex" (Yarrow 1989) — and, perhaps, not that important to save, youth of color may as well be subjected to the horror of safe sex and safe drug use education. This "targeted" education

Fatal Advice

does not transform youth of color into citizens, but instead quarantines them in/as the ground zero of the epidemic.

If white adolescents — future citizens — are unlikely to engage in risk behaviors, youth of color are considered unlikely to change their behavior or escape the environment that marks them as premodern. Whereas white adolescents need neutral information to protect them from initiating drug use and sex out of marriage (i.e., unsafe sex), youth of color are thought to have the nearly impossible task of learning to make sex and drug use safer, but never safe. Thus, AIDS education directed at young people is a component of a broader, racially inflected national pedagogy that includes the war on drugs and the new sexual austerity. The white adolescent serves as the figure to be protected while young people of color, represented as the lower echelon of the drug-selling world, are the figures of social tolerance gone radically awry, simultaneously the victims and the perpetuators of the "broken [black] family."

AIDS Education: Battling the Narratives of Deviant Bodies

By the early 1990s, the reality that persons between the ages of twelve and twenty-one were contracting HIV in alarming numbers was just becoming part of the American consciousness. But this growing acknowledgement (one hates to say *awareness* — how long can a country not know about the 25,000 young people living with AIDS in its schools, hospitals, families, and streets?) of the presence of young people living with AIDS was easily incorporated into existing narratives about sexual development.

As I have shown, larger cultural narratives about the transition to adult sexuality view white, working/middle-class youth as "normally abnormal" for the duration of their adolescence. In popular AIDS discourse, they are at risk if they engage in sex before they achieve the wisdom of conventional adulthood. In stark contrast to this central trope of teen AIDS risk are the gay teenager and the young person of color: for opposite reasons, neither can achieve the safety of adult sexuality. Whereas white working/middle-class adolescents can be protected from HIV if they can be prevented from having sex or experimenting with drugs, gay teens and youth of color are irreversibly and persistently at risk from their nature (the homosexual desires of gay teens) or from their natural environment (the ghetto supposed to harbor all youth of color). White working/middle-class adolescents are presumed unin-fected, gay teens yet to be infected, and youth of color already infected.

The informational and counseling needs of the three groups are perceived to be radically different. While the media suggest that gay youth can learn about safe sex before it is too late, neither the media nor the schools seem prepared to provide such information. Gay teens are left with the sexual equivalent of on-the-job training — simultaneously inaugurating their sexual careers and learning about safe sex. Gay male sex is covertly policed by making it difficult for a young person to get useful information: if he is lucky, he will find an older man to initiate him into the mysteries of safe sex. If not, well, that is the price of membership. The equivocal acknowledgment of gay teens arises only because the confused, uncomfortably queer boy could be-come something worse: the repressed bisexual whose teenage indiscretions threaten to bring HIV into the adult, heterosexual, mainstream society.

Young people of color are considered virtual adults. On one hand, this designation loosened the grip of propriety that had strangled most sexually explicit educational efforts. But on the other hand, because they are so "hard to reach" it is unlikely that funds will be available on an ongoing basis to urban youth projects, already perceived as likely to fail. Gay teens and youth of color may be able to contain risk, but their sex will never be wholly safe. The future possibility of risk (their nature, their environment) always circum-scribes their sexuality. By contrast, white, mainstream heterosexual sexuality is believed always safe until intruded upon by prostitution or bisexuality. Besieged by raging hormones and in a state of temporary insanity, the adoles-cent is at risk only for awhile, elsewhere and from others. Now also at risk from the perversion of safe sex education itself, adolescents need to be steered away from knowledge about safe sex lest it put ideas into their heads about having sex at all.

This logic of who can benefit from what knowledge of safe sex produced a tension between reforming or circumscribing deviant bodies' practice of sex and protecting the "normal" body through anxious silence. This tension, with its necessary assumptions about the relative dispensibility of categories of youth, continues to result in both government inaction and media misrepre-sentation that distract our attention from "where the trouble is": not in the black or gay ghetto but in the hearts and minds of mainstream America.

3

The Erotics of
Innocence

The AIDS epidemic was a shock to America. The vociferous sexual revolution of the 1960s seemed to have drifted into a quiet sexual individualism in the 1970s. America did not quite return to a state of innocence, but most Americans could feel safely distant from sexualities that others might explore. With the onslaught of AIDS, however, as a *Life* magazine cover put it, "No One Is Safe." At least, no one could avoid thinking about AIDS. But as I suggested in chapter 1, the media and public health officials rapidly mobilized two very different ways of and reasons for thinking about AIDS: one for those seen as at risk of contracting HIV and one for those at risk of failing to be compassionate due to their misplaced fears of infection. However, the arbitrariness of social definition on which this split message rested meant that individual Americans did not easily line up behind the risk/compassion distinction. The line separating compassion and risk was so difficult to sustain that the media jumped at any opportunity to reinforce it by using stereotyped and hysterical tales of HIV contagion that defied every fact the citizen had been taught. This chapter explores in detail one such case.

While media coverage of AIDS has continually referred to "innocent victims," the idea of innocence is always relational, performative, and deeply contingent on beliefs about the parties to a possible occasion of transmission. For example, many people outside gay male communities consider gay men fully culpable for their behavior. However, within gay male communities, some individuals are considered less "innocent" than others. People who consider sex between men to be caveat emptor often still consider women to be "innocent" in relationship to those same men. With the exception of Kimberly Bergalis, who was supposed to have been infected by her HIV seropositive dentist's failure to properly sterilize dental equipment, media accounts contain virtually no sustained accounts of the "innocent" victim him- or herself. The infected person was "guilty" unless he or she could "prove" their relative innocence, usually by denying membership in any of the "deviant" groups supposed to be uniquely susceptible to HIV infection. But these denials rarely overcame rumors of secret drug use or sexual misbehavior. No epidemiologically or socially defined group has proven securely "innocent": innocence is an empty category, a state of suspension between the citizenry and the deviants. Those who claimed innocence had to blame their infection on someone deeper in the danger zone, the imaginary hierarchy of people who might "give you AIDS."

By the late 1980s, the "innocent victim" was a well-worn placeholder, a way of imagining someone else who would be less responsible for their plight than the group or individual actually under discussion. The particular individual who was "innocent" for the moment was a sign for a relationship that had breached the line between compassionate citizenship and pitiable deviation. Media accounts often used women to fill this role in juxtaposition to bisexual men. But as I have shown elsewhere (1994), the same media portrayed the individual woman who actually contracts HIV from such a man as "loose" or a dupe who is unable to distinguish "real" men from those who may have contracted HIV from another man. While generally constituted as relatively innocent, the hemophiliac man was not represented as the victim of medical malpractice, but a hostage to his body and its desperate need for supplemental blood components. His wife was relatively *more* innocent, but even she was recast as culpable if she passed HIV to her unborn child. Even babies failed to make the grade as innocent victims. The highly publicized "boarder babies" living with HIV, supposedly abandoned by their drug-using mothers of color, *were* figures of pathos, but like people of color generally, they were considered victims of fate, implicitly responsible for being in the wrong social category. Ultimately, innocence only existed in the abstract: the huge stigma of contracting HIV continued to make every individual person living with the virus suspect of having "done something wrong."

Fatal Advice

Since designating an innocent is opportunistic, even otherwise scary street kids can be converted into victims, but it takes a little more effort: a pedophilic sex monster may be required as their victimizer. The media representation of "Uncle Eddie" Savitz, in which deeply entrenched concepts about sexuality collaborated with ideas about teens' risk for contracting HIV, produced tough, streetwise, young men as the most unlikely victims of a pathetic, upper-class fetishist. Even public health officials believed the culpability machine had stretched the bounds of reasonable science. Nevertheless, the media had its feast, and it was doubly fatal. Eddie Savitz would die under house arrest, only released from jail to a hospice for his final days. The second casualty was the clear explanation of the biomechanics of HIV transmission, crucial as a basis for developing a protective safe sex logic. The media coverage flattened the idea of risk to include any sexual behavior across age lines or with a person living with AIDS.

It is easy to overwhelm what people *know* with what they *fear*. Existing stereotypes quickly amalgamate with misrepresentations of medical and sociological knowledge. Once started, contagion frenzies take on a life of their own. Although some people believe that information can offset fear, cultural narratives of perversion and contagion seem endlessly capable of turning apparently interpretation-proof facts into ammunition for media hysteria and individual discrimination. These morality tales are most volatile when a class of "innocent" victims can be secured as a story's referent. But in the context of a largely sexually transmitted disease, the very notion of innocence is itself constituted by fears and convictions that have little to do with any actual possibility of transmitting an etiologic agent.

A Contagion of Innocence

The most heated exchange came when Abraham [the District Attorney] and city Health Commissioner Robert K. Ross refused to say how many teenage boys had reported having sex with Savitz.

Officials vowed they would never say whether any of those teenagers were found to have contracted AIDS. . . . Ross said it is difficult to ascertain how many teenagers engaged in the highest-risk activity — unprotected anal sex with Savitz.

As reporters tried to get Ross to pinpoint how many youths might have been put at risk of AIDS by their contact with Savitz, the questioning was cut off and Ross was escorted from the podium. . . .

Before he left the podium, however, Ross continued to insist that the potential health threat was not as great as officials, including Abraham, had suggested. (*Philadelphia Inquirer*, April 3, 1992, B1, 3)

On March 25, 1992, "Uncle Eddie" Savitz, a Philadelphia man described by the media as having been diagnosed with AIDS, was arrested for allegedly having sex with some large number of teenage boys. The boys' underage status and the allegation that Savitz had "lied" to one or more boys when asked if he "had AIDS" produced Savitz as a sex monster and the teenagers as innocent victims. Bail was set at $20 million, a figure associated with mass murderers or organized crime figures: Savitz would die under house arrest, never convicted of a crime, never tried on the meager charge of possession of kiddie porn laid against him, and never charged with any act that could have resulted in HIV transmission. The story instantly made CNN and the *New York Times* and was, of course, opulently reported in the *Philadelphia Inquirer* over the next weeks.

As frequently occurs when there is a high-profile AIDS-related story, AIDS hotlines reported a dramatic rise in calls. Some came from Philadelphians who thought they might have had sex with Savitz. But most came from countless others for whom the sensational media coverage and widely reported conflicts between the Public Health Commissioner and the District Attorney raised the specter of their own "innocent" infection from hazily remembered others. Equally unsurprising, violence against gays and others perceived to "have AIDS" reportedly increased, causing another kind of panic among the city's gays and persons living with AIDS.

Legally speaking, "sex charges" covers a wide range of activities, from unwanted touching to rape short of murder. The actual charges against Savitz were not specified for more than a week and, when they were finally enumerated, seemed rather less spectacular than the news coverage had suggested. As reported in the April 3 *Philadelphia Inquirer,* charges appeared to include allegations of contact with only four boys, none of whom would testify to having joined Savitz in anal intercourse, the major HIV transmission-enabling sexual behavior between men. In addition, prosecutors were said to be preparing the following evidence: photographs of Savitz in "sexually suggestive poses with two fifteen-year-old boys" allegedly taken on the day of his arrest; testimony by one of those boys that Savitz "asked to have oral sex with him that day"; a second boy's statement that Savitz had "performed oral sex on him about nine times since September, when the boy was fourteen"; another statement by a seventeen-year-old boy who said Savitz photographed him and "paid him to let Savitz perform oral sex on him between 1989 and 1991"; and, finally, "a roommate's statement that Savitz told him 'he had oral and anal sex' with an unspecified number of some five hundred boys that the roommate says visited Savitz since 1989." Police also claimed to have a deposition from a single boy, aged fifteen, who said he had anal intercourse with Savitz "an unspecified number of times," but there was no indication whether the boy was the recipient or inserter, nor whether condoms had been used. In the same *Inquirer* account, defense attorneys were reported as stating that the police reports they had been given contained no mention of anal intercourse and "dispute that this man engaged in any intrusive sexual activity that wasn't protected."

From the first day's coverage, when Savitz was said to have had sex with countless Philadelphia "boys," to the ultimate enumeration of the charges, it appeared that most of the "contact" between Savitz and the boys consisted in his fellating the boys (from the standpoint of HIV transmission, constituting no risk to the boys). What seemed to upset some people was that Savitz had purchased boys' soiled underwear and feces samples, which he reportedly collected in separate, labeled pizza boxes. Irrespective of the biology of transmission, the fact that a person living with AIDS was indicted on underage sex charges of any kind prompted panic that hundreds, perhaps thousands of Philadelphia's male youth had been "exposed to AIDS."

Panic over the form of Savitz's sexual interests colluded with panic over AIDS generally to override the display of even minimal accuracy regarding the basics of HIV transmission. The *Inquirer*'s editorial slip — "highest-risk activity — anal intercourse with Savitz" — quite baldly displayed the underlying belief that any association with Savitz, much less "contact," meant contagion. The news stories provide no good reason to believe that Savitz wasn't practicing safe sex. But that hardly mattered: if HIV was not transmitted then perversion itself might be. Ironically, though, since intercourse, irrespective of gender, age, or other object choice attribute, is the most dangerous form of sex from the standpoint of HIV transmission, it was the very dispersion of Savitz's sexual aim into scopophilia, fetishism, and oral servicing that provided the boys' safety from HIV infection.

The Danger of Innocence

Savitz's arrest and detention until his death from an HIV complication (he was begrudgingly released to a hospice for his final days) raise important political and theoretical issues about the pop psychology that undergirds media representation and, tragically for Edward Savitz, legal argumentation. The panic that killed Savitz was grounded in a series of confusions: adolescents were constituted as intrinsically innocent objects of desire; HIV was conflated with AIDS; and the psychoanalytic distinction between sexual object and sexual aim and their relation to deviations or perversions was lost.

Together, these slippages engendered one category — "sexual contact" — comprised of at least two. The first set — scopophilia, fetishism, and fellatio — are only dangerous from the standpoint of cultural fears of sexual difference, while the second category, intercourse, is dangerous from the standpoint of HIV infection. Combining "perverse" sex with a "normal" person and "normal" sex with a pervert under the label "dangerous" ignores the requirements for HIV transmission. This conflation leads directly to fear of *any* sexualized contact with supposed deviants — especially if they are thought to be living with AIDS — while ignoring the hazards of "normal" sex with "normal" individuals — presumed uninfected with HIV. The problematic split, already articulated as the national pedagogy, generated such a huge national media frenzy because Savitz's sexual objects were teenage boys who, despite being tough and streetwise, and because they were refugees from the white working and middle classes, could still be recruited to the category of innocence.

As described in chapter 2, youth is a malleable term that has been divided into three connotative categories in AIDS discourse. Adolescent *innocence* is an even more unstable category, one that adults produce by combining the nostalgia for a time before sexual knowledge with the presumption that children desire to become adult, that is, sexual. As I showed in chapter 2, the adolescent's sexual stirring foretells but does not produce the sexual subject/adult. Adulthood is accomplished through sexual practice, when it is understood as such.

In early psychoanalytic theory, innocence was crafted from two forms of memory, or rather, *lack* of memory: first, as Sigmund Freud describes cultural beliefs about virginity, "The demand that the girl shall bring with her into marriage with one man no memory of sexual relations with another is after all nothing but a logical consequence of the exclusive right of possession over a woman which is the essence of monogamy — it is but an extension of this monopoly onto the past" (1963: 70). The second lack of memory creates a situation in which adults are trapped in the moment just after innocence has been lost. Under analysis, the adult's neuroses are linked to a desire to recapture the time, now ever receding, before which the mother was recognized as sexual. The adult becomes sure that this moment existed but can never recall it, hence, it must be perpetually reinvented as a surplus: the adult clings to and disavows sexual knowledge as the mirror memory of innocence lost.[1]

Thus, innocence, and those who break cultural taboo by overtly staking their erotic life on it, is a gnomon, a space left over after the production of sexual memory. Innocence should remain unspoken and is unspeakable, but the erotic practices that circulate around the articulation of innocence and the complex social institutions designed to protect it each chip away at the space of innocence. They demand to know whether innocence knows what it is, they forcibly disqualify the innocent by pressing him or her into the production of a narrative about innocence that is always, or becomes, retrospective, about innocence lost. Innocence is, in the first instance, actually linked with rather than opposed to sexual knowledge.

Discussions of innocence usually concern the acquisition of knowledge about sex in the transition from childhood to adulthood. But in AIDS discourse, notions of innocence take on a legal quality, involving questions pertaining to the right to withhold information ("lie," "protect confidentiality") about HIV serostatus, and from whom. In the late 1980s, for the most part, adult sex was caveat emptor; people *ought* to tell you their serostatus and sexual history, but you couldn't really count on their doing so. In a few cases, the failure to inform a coparticipant in unprotected sex was used as a basis for criminal charges. Usually, however, the indicted person was already considered predatory — a prostitute, African national, or queer of some variety. All of these cases are remarkable for trying to construct HIV seropositives as willfully infecting others (for revenge) or willfully disregarding the potential harm to others.

The exception to this structured innocence was wives, but not unmarried female partners, of bisexual men. Single women are supposed to realize that any of their male partners might have had sex with men, but the vows of matrimony are premised on spousal honesty. This belief about the marital contract complicated the already difficult debates about whether states should institute contact-tracing programs for people who test positive for the HIV antibody. While most states offer voluntary contact-tracing programs, some states have passed laws enabling physicians to contact partners if they believe the HIV antibody positive person will not do so. The major argument lodged in these cases is that because of the furtive nature of male bisexuals (as opposed to their better adjusted, "open" gay peers) they will not tell their wives about their sex lives or serostatus, if they discover themselves seropositive.

Thus, innocence is bound up not only in knowledge about sex but also in perceptions of who is required to learn about their serostatus, and who has the right to discover someone else's. Most of the categories of people who are thought of as at risk are also thought responsible for figuring out whether they have been infected. A few — largely white middle-class women whom the national pedagogy shielded from explicit knowledge about their own and their partners' potential for risk — may have their innocence destroyed by a physician who breaks the bad news that they are now infected.

These debates about contact tracing and innocence complicated the Savitz case since he was alleged to have answered no when asked if he had AIDS. Savitz may have been playing semantics, despite suspecting that the boy who made this allegation was concerned more about infection than Savitz's failing health. Or, he may have answered truthfully enough: he was apparently symptomatic, but the AIDS definition at the time of his case was highly restrictive. Savitz may not yet have carried that diagnosis. Whatever occurred in that complex exchange of information, what Savitz said is no more a "lie" than the media's reproduction of the confused allegation. No one is served by confusing the distinction between HIV and AIDS.

Most scientists now believe that HIV, along with a potentially wide variety of cofactors, is the principal, but not sufficient, etiologic agent that may, some ten years after infection, result in immune system failure sufficient to render the infected person susceptible to the many opportunistic infections, cancers, or changes in body function that bring with them an AIDS diagnosis. Although measurable changes and some debilitating infections occur within a few years after infection, in the majority of cases opportunistic infections or the generalized direct effects of HIV (generalized failure to thrive and some forms of encephalopathy) occur after the crucial T-4 cells drop from the normal eight to twelve hundred parts per milliliter to less than two hundred, losing, in the majority of cases, an average about one hundred parts each year after infection. With prophylaxis now available for *pneumocystis carinii* pneumonia (PCP), once the major cause of death in people diagnosed with AIDS, a significant number of people who have been infected for a long time (ten to fifteen years) live with negligible T-cell counts. But until early 1993, when the Centers for Disease Control adopted a new criterion, they did not qualify for an AIDS diagnosis. HIV-infected individuals can presumably be infectious for a decade or more — though to varying degrees — before recognizable symptoms occur. These evolving diagnostic nuances have left relatively asymptomatic but long-infected people in doubt about whether — or on what day, and by whose decree — they "have AIDS." Thus, asking whether someone "has AIDS" is not very helpful for those who insist on grounding partner selection in medical histories. While asking whether someone has tested positive for the HIV antibody might seem more specific, it is likely that many people just don't know, or prefer not to tell, and instead simply engage exclusively in risk-eliminating behavior or consider it their partners' duty to ask for safe sex. The question was a bad one, but, as I have shown, the insistence on using serostatus as a means of choosing partners was at the heart of the 1980s partner selection strategy: the media reports of the Savitz case used this fatal advice as if it were the basis of criminal law.

Viral Monstrosity

Like the stories of Ryan White or Ali Geertz, the Savitz story might have provided the national pedagogy with an occasion for a lesson in compassion. Far from providing an occasion for compassion, the Savitz coverage actually untaught some key information that health educators consider to be crucial in helping the public understand why they need not fear widespread contagion, in decreasing fatalism about preventing HIV transmission to oneself, and in improving the situation of already infected people by encouraging them to take advantage of life-prolonging and quality-of-life enhancing measures (Aggleton et al. 1989: 57–59). In the Savitz story, any contact with Savitz is represented as potentially risky. But no one "gets AIDS" through just *any* form of contact; rather, one contracts HIV through specific, known, and relatively difficult routes — sexual intercourse in which there is ejaculation into the anus or vagina; inoculation, either through transfusion or other use of blood products, or through reusing hypodermic needles during medical or nonmedical procedures; and from mother to fetus. The mechanics of infection *to* an inserting partner in "penile" or "manual" intercourse, *to* the receiving partner in either fellatio or cunnilingus, or *to* a partner in contact with menstrual blood are still in dispute, with the numbers of U.S. cases attributed to each of these routes anecdotal or very low.

In the Savitz case, the confusion between HIV and AIDS was all the more remarkable because only five months earlier, during Magic Johnson's November 1991 revelation of his positive HIV serostatus, the same news sources had gone out of their way to explain the crucial distinction. Recruiting Johnson as a narrative device for explaining AIDS to consumers of news media was apparently successful: in the methadone clinics where I was working at the time, it was not unusual for clients to describe HIV as "what Magic's got" — as opposed to AIDS. If Magic Johnson was to operate as a lesson in virology and as a wholesome role model to young people, he had to be produced as (still) a figure of health and strength who simply hadn't heeded the warnings soon enough. Black youths were supposed to identify with Magic and heed his warning. But Savitz was not allowed a heroic side — he did not offer advice, but was the very image of the creature young people were warned *about*. For Savitz to play the role of monster in relation to street teens (elsewhere represented as the people against whom "adolescents" should be protected), he had to be produced as always and already sick, even before he acquired HIV. Indeed, as a pervert, he might even have "it" (them? . . . HIV? homosexuality?) sui generis. If the careful coverage of Magic Johnson's HIV status momentarily taught a nation the difference between HIV and AIDS, the very same media's coverage of Savitz set HIV education back many years.

Habeas Corpus: CNN's "Boy"

By 1992, media consumers were accustomed to associating sexual danger with the one-way exchange of pernicious bodily fluids from "carriers" to "innocent victims." Gay male to gay male sexual transmission and junkie to junkie needle-sharing transmission were considered victimless acts, side effects of deviant subcultures that people entered with their eyes open. However, both bisexual men *and* drug injectors were considered carriers who intentionally infected women through "ordinary" heterosexual intercourse, or by luring white, middle-class adolescent thrill seekers into their lifestyle. Women sex workers were described as acquiring HIV through drug injection even while they supposedly willfully infect their johns during sex, denying the reality that women, including sex workers, are at substantially greater risk *from* men during condomless heterosexual intercourse.

Schooled in this system of tropes, readers of the Savitz story had to exert a certain amount of labor to decode and interpret the exchange of money for dry if soiled underwear as dangerous sex. So, CNN came up with a body. The principal "boy" interviewed on CNN, a big, tough-talking youth, casually stated that it was widely known on the streets that young men could make a few easy bucks off Uncle Eddie. In the young man's account, Uncle Eddie was benign; if anything, viewers who followed the case got the impression that his fetish for soiled youthful underwear made Savitz something of a victim to the young hustler's mercantile schemes. Nevertheless, CNN offered the boy's account as evidence of Savitz's potential for rampant HIV transmission.

The CNN boy punctuated the Savitz story in two ways. First, he reminded viewers that adolescents are supposedly sexually liminal, possessing (or possessed by) sexual desires but not yet engaging in fully sexual acts (i.e., intercourse) understood as such. Especially in regard to the selling of underwear, the boy seemed not to register Savitz's oddities as *sexual:* part of the danger of teens' liminal sexualities is that they may inadvertently engage in behaviors that they do not "know" are "sex," as they will later recognize it as an adult. But second, because of his innocence, the boy triggered the logic that *required* public exposure of Savitz's serostatus. Despite the failure to establish a plausible route of HIV transmission between Savitz and the boys (much less *their* serostatus), the boy symbolized the possibility of obtaining legal proof of Savitz's guilt as a sex murderer.

In order to secure the interpretive grid within which viewers could per-ceive Savitz's monstrosity, the media elaborated on several cultural beliefs about adolescent sexuality. Whereas Savitz's perversions (homosexuality, pedophilia, scopophilia, a fixation on oral servicing) signified a derailed sex-ual trajectory, the boy's participation could be explained away as an innocent, if hazardous, phase. Part of the difficulty faced by CNN's interviewer was that he couldn't really ask the boy too much lest he provoke the boy's sexual self-recognition. Thus, the interview performs the divide between adults and ado-lescents: adults are subjects because they recognize their sexuality even if they are embarrassed to speak of it. Adolescents hover at the fateful line where to speak of sexuality is to evidence sexuality, to introject it into an otherwise innocent body. This broad paradox has meant that the supposed victims of sex crimes, in order to convict their violators and preserve the sanctity of innocence in general (the victim's is now lost), must tell authorities what happened; they must narrate from the standpoint of a sexual subject. But to confess the crime committed against them means they have knowledge, a memory, which, de facto, means they are no longer an innocent.

To make the innocent speak produces their sexual experiences as a narra-tive, a text too close to the voyeurism and snapshot pornography that both the police and CNN had considered tantamount to sex. But CNN found a novel solution to the problem of producing evidence against Savitz without par-ticipating in sexualizing the boy. Unlike the accused, but not yet prosecuted, Savitz, whose gentle if slightly troubled face was recognizable in any house-hold reached by CNN, the boy's image was digitally obscured. The legal presumption that Savitz would be innocent until proven guilty is undercut by the evidentiary boy whose natural innocence serves as a prohibition to repre-senting him. Thus, the boy "speaks" without a face. CNN's faceless teenager at risk of contracting HIV was consistent with the media's general representa-tion of teens and AIDS.

The ambivalently sexual, not-quite-adult *body* was invoked, but, like the media generally, CNN declined to put a "face" on young people who might be at risk. The persistent problematic of the gnomon space of innocence sent AIDS education and policy in the wrong direction during the crucial mid-1980s, when young people, especially young people of color and young gay men, were being diagnosed with AIDS with no real recognition of the fact that they could contract HIV. Youth of the 1980s heard plenty about not discriminating against people living with AIDS, but learned virtually nothing useful about how to prevent themselves from entering that category.

Object and Aim

As I suggested in the last chapter, the national pedagogy was structured around the general belief in adolescence — even given variations by gender, ethnicity, and geography — as a time of turmoil between a period of innocence (childhood) and one of accomplished identity and safety (adulthood). The "storm and stress" theory is the default mode for policy advocates and AIDS researchers, who produce adolescence as a stage, however difficult to pin down, during which young people are exposed to features of a previously unavailable adult lifestyle, but without the necessary skills to actually operate responsibly as adults. Even when actively engaged in supposedly adult-defining behaviors (sexual intercourse and drug injection), adolescents somehow perform with childish attitudes, with a lack of full understanding of what they are doing. Adolescent risk taking is explained away: teens are described as incapable of judging the future consequences of current acts and as believing they are immortal. While much of the data researchers offer bear out these conclusions, it is unclear that most adults are any better at looking to their future or evaluating the consequences of proximate risks. Apparently, adults are allowed to choose self-destructive behaviors (alcohol consumption, cigarette smoking, eating a bad diet, and overwork) that would count as impaired adolescent reasoning if engaged in by a slightly younger person.

This particular construction of adolescents as unbalanced and on the cusp of acting without full understanding underlies the confusion in the Savitz accounts concerning sexual object and aim. In the early twentieth century, Freud introduced two terms in hopes of clarifying different priorities or axes of sexuality: "The person from whom sexual attraction proceeds [is] the *sexual object* and the act toward which the instinct tends [is] the *sexual aim*" (1963: 1–2). The Savitz coverage, and accounts of adolescence generally, assume adolescence to be a time of deflected object and aim. They define adulthood as the point after which object and aim are fixed, even if the adult fixes on an object of the "wrong" gender. It is critical to mark this dual aspect of sexuality: adolescents may engage in either wrong-object or nonintercourse activities without being "deviants." Only adults who persist in selecting the wrong object or aim (or both, in the case of homosexuals who did what the nation asked and stopped engaging in intercourse) are considered deviant. But the extent to which deviations of object and deviations of aim are seen as problematic varies and, in fact, changed during the 1980s under pressure from safe sex discourse, on one side (which argues for deviation of aim), and right-wing backlash (which rails against deviation of object), on the other.

The apparent decrease in homophobia evident in opinion polls of the late 1980s and popular discourse about AIDS generally accepts homosexual object choice as valid or at least workable, that is, susceptible to change toward safer sex. But this only occurred because the popular history of gay male sexuality was analogized to the same trajectory from innocence to intercourse that I have been describing here and in chapter 2. The sexual revolution of the 1970s was equated with the meaningless play of burgeoning desires and the inability to foresee future dire consequences thought to characterize the individual adolescent. As two early AIDS commentators (Fettner and Check 1984) describe it: "the realities of AIDS may turn [gay men's] inchoate desires into a political consensus. . . . Gay men are being forced by AIDS to reorganize their personal priorities, to put aside self-preoccupation and to turn their abilities outward to the good of a wider community" (243). This description suggests that acceptance of homosexuality occurred because an adult gay community characterized by altruism, political participation, and, tacitly, safe sex emerged. But anytime we notice a change in views about homosexuality we must also ask whether there has been a shift in the underlying calculus of object and aim: the high cost of the citizen's refusal to acknowledge their own potential risk was the legitimation of a homosexual *object* for the aim — intercourse — that the national pedagogy refused to challenge more generally.

A 1990 *Newsweek* feature on "The Future of Gay America," which de-scribed a party in which "5,000 condoms rained down on guests" (22) in a nightclub — the "encouraging sign that safe sex works" (23) — used the now worn device of signifying safe sex through the mention of condoms. This persistent focus on condoms and their association with the new gay male sexuality of the AIDS era — "infection among gay men has been dropping since 1987" (*Newsweek* 1990: 23) — insisted that intercourse, the riskiest practice, was to be the mature and stable form of homosexual sex, the ideo-logically "safe" deviation.

The growing belief in intercourse as *the* mark of adult homosexuality is recent, perhaps an effect of the national pedagogy's reluctance to elaborate safe sex. Reviewing early sexological findings, Freud stated that homosexual men and women had a deviation both of object and of aim (1963: 11–12), that is, they liked members of their gender, but had no interest in having intercourse with them. Freud believed that men prefer manual sex (recirculated as the "mutual masturbation" of AIDS education, a persistently and insidiously demeaning name that reinforces the view of male homosexuality as a projective narcissism) and women wanted to kiss.

Whether this actually reflected any kind of numerical reality is impossible to determine, and there are certainly celebrated cases of "sodomy" involving both lesbians and gay men that would have come to Freud's attention. Indeed, Henry Abelove (1992) argues that the dominance of intercourse as both the preferred method of sexual encounter and the act definitive of "real" sex around which "foreplay" and even "homosexual" acts were organized arose quite late in the modern period and in tandem with the differentiation of work from leisure time. The need to organize sex in order to make room for work may have unconsciously motivated both the insistence on intercourse as the proper aim and sexologists' use of male-female intercourse as the standard alongside which their favored "deviations" coexisted as "normal" "abnormalities."

Under the pressure of safe sex education in the context of AIDS, a homosexuality that was once doubly deviant has now "straightened out" its aim. Now homosexuality and heterosexuality differ only in gender of object choice and in their need for condoms: in the context of this new understanding of gay male sexuality, Savitz was a "deviant" homosexual. With no popular idea of homosexual safe sex other than condomized intercourse, the citizen had no idea how Savitz might make his sex safe. Paradoxically, because he showed little interest in intercourse, the police and media considered him more, not less, likely to infect others.

Contact or Contract? Eddie's "Boys"

Initial accounts claimed that Savitz might have had "sexual contact" with hundreds, thousands, perhaps even five thousand "boys" over the previous three years. These figures, it turned out, were based on police estimates of the number of erotic photographs of purportedly teenage boys confiscated from Savitz's apartment, only some much smaller number of which were photographs in which Savitz himself appeared.

Some portion of the market in erotic photographs of apparently youthful males in fact feature underage models, but many use "adult" models to *represent* "boys." The uncertainty about the actual age of males appearing in pornography has in part fueled the hysteria over "kiddie porn";[2] in order to make it clear that "boys" are being misused, it has been necessary to foreground the very youngest, clearest examples of underage models. Debates about the production of pornography in general have been equivocal about the models' agency in their labor. While adult males and porn venture capitalists undeniably have greater economic and social power than their female and young models, it is significant that antiporn activists and public officials generally treat young models as victims of sexual molestation, not as workers subjected to unfair labor practices. Their sexuality, rather than their role in commercial production, inspires the impulse to protect; apparently there can be no consent to this form of modeling, and such arrangements fall outside labor practice discourse.

In a culture obsessed with youth, it should be no surprise that young men could be imagined as sexual objects. Likewise, in a culture replete with complex systems of representation, especially representations of sexuality, it should be no surprise that low-production-value (pseudo-snapshot) photos of ersatz boys should constitute some percentage of the wares designed to satisfy scopophilic desires. Snapshot porn, which one might have taken oneself, suggests the innocence of the domestic setting. As an object, such photographs enable the invention of a memory of having been accidentally caught in a playful moment with/as an innocent lad.

But both the police and media treated Savitz's photographs as documentation of Savitz's exploits rather than recognizing them as the fetish objects that they palpably were. Savitz's scopophilia was instantly and seamlessly converted into "sexual contact," which, despite the content of the photos (which the *Inquirer* described as "erotic poses," by which they seem to have meant either foreplay or postcoital boasting), was assumed to be evidence of intercourse. Because the police were intent on convicting Savitz, they forgot about the biomechanics of HIV transmission; they failed to recognize voyeurism as a sexual aim distinct from the aim of intercourse. The photographs and underwear collections were treated as trophies: the media and district attorney seemed unable to imagine a sexuality in which intercourse was not the finale.

Work and Sex

Modernity's complex linking of sex and work complicates models of adolescence. Campaigns for child labor laws and mandatory school attendance, which serve the evolving economic needs of industrial and postindustrial societies, have usually been couched in terms of preserving childhood and adolescence as a time free from adult pressures, such as work and sex. These campaigns, and current constructions of youth, presume that the adolescent does not own his or her body; despite their occupation of it, in neither sex nor work can an adolescent legitimately use, improve, wear out, or destroy their body as he or she elects. Adolescence ends only when the body becomes a legitimate vessel of work and sex. This dual aspect of modern adolescence complicates the Savitz case: if Savitz was supposed to have stolen the boys' innocence through premature sex, the CNN boy's casual suggestion that a *lot* of boys knew they could make money from Savitz established the presence of an extensive and calculating underground economy of teenaged, fetish-peddling entrepreneurs.

Media accounts of young people trading sex for money often cast them and their innocence as doubly lost. First, they have sex "prematurely" because they are driven by a need for remunerative work. But having had sex, they develop an adult desire for both more sex and more money. Having sex and achieving economic independence vie for premier place in establishing boys' adulthood. But in the Savitz case, to see these boys as adults because of their commercial ventures implies that they have consented to their transactions, which makes them responsible (as adults) for ensuring the safety of their own sexual activity.

There are significant and gendered consequences to these losses of innocence; selling sex is understood differently in young women than in young men. For young men, hustling is a preliminary form of entrepreneurship. The fact of having sold one's body to men does not imply that the entrepreneur is homosexual. The innocence lost pertains to work; he is no longer a work virgin, but not yet a sexually identifiable item. For a young woman, however, prostitution acts as a nonlegitimate replacement for the culturally sanctioned barter of matrimony. She loses her sexual innocence but maintains her work innocence. She ends up very much defined as a sexual object, not as an entrepreneurial subject. His work serves as a transition to adulthood. Hers eliminates the easiest route to becoming a proper wife and mother.

Teaching or Practicing?

The national pedagogy has actively enlisted adults in the effort to teach safe sex, especially, in promoting partner selection over condoms. This recruitment to pedagogy is duplicitous: first, it saves parents embarrassment by allowing them to discuss partners instead of penises, as for example, in the *Good Housekeeping* (1990) column (discussed in chapter 2), which emphasizes that parents should "make it clear how important it is to select a partner carefully" (257) — but provides no clear advice to parents on how to skirt the issue of sex while warning their children about its dangers. But second, in order to avoid admitting to the possibility of incest, it positions adults as safe and detached givers of advice. The obverse seems to be that any adult who has sex with an underage person must *also* be practicing unsafe sex. This positioning of adults made Eddie Savitz's relation to his boys even more monstrous: instead of personifying the avuncular nation, instead of teaching compassion like a *proper* person living with AIDS, Uncle Eddie "exchanged" money for the boy's body fluids. While he enacted the most fundamental edict of safe sex — conserving body fluids through use of condoms or avoidance of intercourse — he violated the most basic belief underlying the "know your partner" ethos: people living with HIV should not have sex.

In order to teach his boys as they practiced their mutual deviation of aim, Eddie-as-Uncle had to communicate across the vast information divide that was constituted by the national pedagogy. As I suggested in chapter 1, most of the advice that is circulated outside the gay community suggests avoiding sex with persons with HIV and is based upon a "knowledge" about the other that is to be obtained through questioning, proof of antibody status, or guesswork. This advice, directed to heterosexuals in particular, subtly links deviance and seropositivity, suggesting that any sex act is safe with a person known to be HIV antibody negative, while no act is safe (only saf*er*) with a person of unknown or positive antibody status. This advice pointedly ignores a huge number of always safe activities — voyeurism, intercourse with dildos, manual stimulation, etc. — because they are viewed as perversions, as not properly (hetero)*sexual.* One cannot learn about these practices without having lost one's innocence: knowledge of *those* safe activities must be gained through illegitimate channels. In order to vilify Eddie, his boys' calculated participation in a perverse sexual economy must be distinguished from their failure to avoid a person living with AIDS; they are tacitly heterosexualized, placed in the domain of citizen-like avoidance strategies, lacking any knowledge of nonintercourse sexual activities. By applying the citizen's calculus of avoidance, which predicates "safe sex" on the "honesty" of one's partner, Savitz's "lie" seals his production as contagious monster. Savitz's scopophilic and fetishistic protection of the boys cannot be read as safe sex, but as the most egregious form of sexual predation, punishable by death.

Remarkably, there was no suggestion in the Savitz stories that the boys might be gay. They had to be considered straight in order to be counted as victims. Young people are generally considered heterosexuals, even as they "explore" homosexuality. One *works* at homosexuality, while heterosexuality, it seems, comes without practice. Thus, while Eddie was represented as a marginalized homosexual (the "roommate" who was to testify against him, as well as reports of equivocation among gay spokespersons, shore up this idea), the boys were not. Their mutual sexual activity might be described as homosexual, but the boys were "innocent." Their decision-making capacities were presumed to operate in the heterosexual, information-sparse, know-your-partner episteme. Eddie, on the other hand, operated in the homosexual, information-dense, always-practice-safe-sex episteme. In this complex of different quantities of available information and different strategies for arriving at decisions about safe sex, the source of a fall from innocence and the presumption of having, and having to share, knowledge fell on Savitz. Not only did he know (or, as a member of a "risk group," was thought responsible to find out) his HIV serostatus,[3] but he also, ironically, occupied the position of pedagogue, as even the boys, who called him "Uncle" Eddie, recognized. He was thought responsible for conveying knowledge about safe sex, which the innocent young men were presumed unable to have obtained from their families, schools, or leisure activities.

Not one account suggested that Savitz failed to *teach* his boys about safe sex. But, unsurprisingly, not one account suggests that he did. Instead, the news media turned away from the evidence they themselves offered: opulent discussions of many activities that were safe for the boys — being fellated, participating as objects of voyeurism, providing scat for Savitz's complex fetish. Reporters and, apparently, the district attorney persistently failed to make good on the claim that Savitz was *ever* the insertive, but condomless, partner in anal intercourse. Rumors still abound in Philadelphia, but, since Savitz died in custody before he could be tried on the meager underage sex charges (he was never charged with transmitting HIV), no legal definition of safe sex could be culled from this case. The insistence on blurring age of consent laws with the emerging case law relating to reckless endangerment by having unprotected intercourse (a charge that has rarely been successful even as a sentence enhancement, adult "consent" being prized above all) testifies to the national pedagogy's refusal to designate any nonintercourse, nonheterosexual sex activities as *safe*. Apparently, American culture prefers to police its narrow boundaries rather than allowing young people to imagine any other sex than the single form that, from the standpoint of HIV transmission, is the most dangerous.

AIDS Panics/AIDS Education

Sensational AIDS contagion stories consolidate hazardous cultural logics, but do not produce them sui generis. The Savitz feeding frenzy undid any gains made during the Magic Johnson coverage and, far from alerting Philadelphians to the dangers (or safety) of HIV-carrying, pedophilic fetishists, increased confusion about sexuality and blurred the important distinction between HIV and AIDS, which in turn decreased the opportunities for providing useful advice to young people. Most safe sex education, and media coverage like that surrounding the Savitz case, constitutes intercourse as *the* identity-conveying adult sexual act while it simultaneously increases anxiety about protecting the "innocent." This feature of national AIDS pedagogy seems to promote the most risk-enabling act while at the same time issuing a gag order on explaining how to do it safely. As long as the responsibility for "causing"

HIV infection is laid at the door of the people with whom teenagers may have sex, the "know your partner" strategy will prevail. It will be promoted over strategies like condoms or the far-from-innocent choice of other pleasurable nonintercourse activities.

Cultural notions of innocence dovetail with notions of risk and are differentially constructed by gay versus straight cultures. At least on the ideological level most urban gay men seem to accept that they will have to use condoms in order to engage in intercourse: a significant portion simply always have safe sex without revealing or inquiring about serostatus. Their heterosexual cohorts, by contrast, continue to trust in their own capacity to distinguish the innocent from the complicit, that is, they continue to believe in innocence. They develop ever more complex schemes for quizzing their partners or looking for signs of danger.

As long as innocence is differentially distributed, the apparent need for changes in sexual practices will be differentially distributed. But curbing HIV transmission might require that everyone change their sexual practices. However, the changes in concepts of homosexual practice both inside and outside the gay community, as well as the emergence of a strongly felt sense of "heterosexual" identity among young Americans, helped the citizen avoid confronting this possibility. Freud was sure that inverts were doubly perverse, in both object and aim. A century later we may find that deviations of aim are a survival tactic, and gay men, no longer innocent and having normalized safe sex, may provide the best model for self-conscious, ingenious sexual development.

The fatal divide between the citizen's and the deviant's concepts of safe sex increased through the 1980s, especially as gay men educated themselves about the science and sexual politics of the epidemic. While America was busy mounting a national pedagogy that exiled deviance but sacrificed its youth, gay men of all ages pursued safe sex education, which was sometimes underwritten by the desire to be accepted as "responsible citizens," even if infected. But there was a persistent dissidence that rejected the proliferation of information and the objectification of sexuality it entailed. The next two chapters describe the trajectory of safe sex as an activism that was finally antinational and understood to be obscene by those administering the national pedagogy.

The Erotics of Innocence

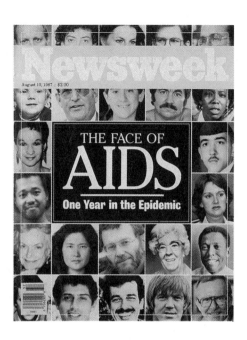

August 10, 1987 : $2.00

THE FACE OF
AIDS
One Year in the Epidemic

(*Above and opposite*) *Newsweek* simultaneously applauded its own objectivity and unabashedness and invented the idea of compassion in its August 10, 1987 cover story that put "the real face" on AIDS. The opening editorial, accompanied by reproductions of the seven previous covers featuring stories about AIDS, explains: "The acronym AIDS was still a frightening new word in the American lexicon when *Newsweek* published its first cover report on the epidemic in April 1983 — one of the earliest in any mainstream publication. Subsequent cover stories have tracked the search for causes and cures; have examined the impact of the disease on American society and particularly on gay men, its most numerous casualties; and have followed an AIDS doctor and his team on their rounds among the sick and dying. But this week's 16-page Special Report, the magazine's eighth AIDS cover in four years, reaches past the numbers and the epidemiological charts to focus on the human cost of the illness. It is the photo journal of a plague year — a gallery of 302 men, women and children struck down by the epidemic in the 12 months ending last

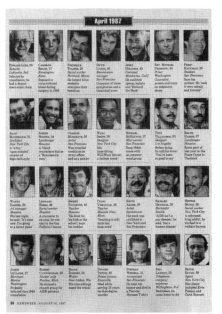
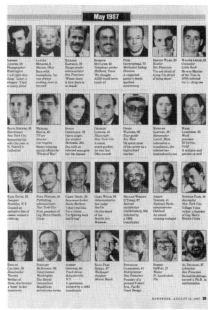

week. They range in age from an infant of one to a widow of 87, and they come from every walk of life from mailman to banker, from housewife to superstar. To look into their mostly young eyes is to see the real fact of AIDS" (p. 3).

Although the relentless march of faces was moving, even to the most bitter activist, the faces were, finally, a parade. The compression into the phrase "the Face of AIDS" of the lives, hopes, foibles, and, yes, faces of the many, many people infected with HIV or diagnosed with AIDS did the opposite of personalizing the tragedy: it collapsed a disease into substitutable bodies — *individual people* — who were now visually spectacular examples of the stereotypes of people citizens might fear or pity.

85

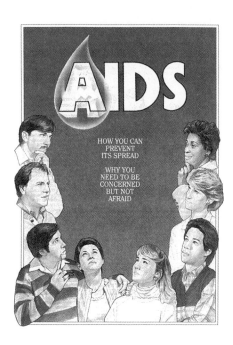

(*Above and opposite*) This colorful 1988 pamphlet emphasizes tolerance and reasonableness. Outlining the shift from scare tactics to the invention of a compassionate citizen who is extremely unlikely to be at risk, the pamphlet explains "why everyone needs to be concerned . . . but not afraid": "AIDS. It's a chilling disease that has already taken the lives of thousands of people. . . . AIDS has the potential to affect everyone — ourselves, our families, and our friends. Still, some people remain indifferent to the facts. Some are unaware that they may be putting themselves at risk; other may be unnecessarily afraid of getting AIDS through casual, everyday contact. But by learning the truth about AIDS, we will be able to stop worrying about the wrong things, and protect ourselves from the true risks" (p. 2).

Typically, there are no strangers, only people we know, in this kinder, gentler, visually multiethnic (and even queer!) America. But however utopian the approach taken by Krames Communications, it leaves several important features of the pamphlet's logic unexplained. Who is responsible for the "lies" that this "truth" will unmask — militant homosexuals or the government? What exactly are the "true risks" — acts or attitudes?

at work, or while eating in a restaurant; nor are children at risk at school. Knowing this, we can begin to really understand that it is risky behavior we should be wary of, not the person with AIDS. We can do much to help protect others—from the disease, the fear, and the suffering—through sharing what we have learned and showing we care.

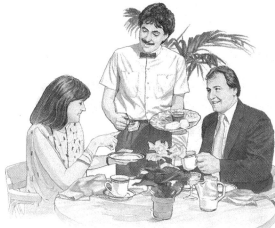

The AIDS virus is not spread in food, or on eating utensils such as dishes, cups, knives, and forks.

In the Community
Experts agree that the AIDS virus is not spread during casual social situations. You don't have to worry, for example, if a food preparer or server has AIDS. Or about getting AIDS from eating utensils, drinking fountains, bathrooms, swimming pools, or gym equipment. Sitting next to someone in a crowded bus or train is not a risk for AIDS transmission either.

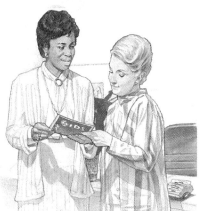

You Can Make the Difference
You can start today to help stop the spread of AIDS as well as the unnecessary fear and suffering. Help educate others—including children and teenagers—about AIDS. Share the information about low-risk behaviors, and reassure them that AIDS is not spread by casual contact. Practice low-risk behavior if your lifestyle might expose you to the virus. Show you care by contributing time or money to support AIDS research and education. And if at some point a friend or colleague has the disease, treat him or her with compassion—not fear.

If we ignore AIDS until one of our friends or family becomes infected, it will be too late. Prevent AIDS by spreading the facts—not the fear.

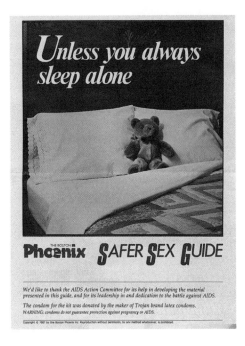

Unless you always sleep alone

Phœnix ▪ SAFER SEX GUIDE

We'd like to thank the AIDS Action Committee for its help in developing the material presented in this guide, and for its leadership and dedication to the battle against AIDS.

The condom for the kit was donated by the maker of Trojan brand latex condoms.

WARNING: condoms do not guarantee protection against pregnancy or AIDS.

Copyright © 1987 by the Boston Phoenix Inc. Reproduction without permission, by any method whatsoever, is prohibited.

The hip weekly *Boston Phoenix* struggled to produce as its audience people who should practice safer sex. Interestingly the advice on the "menu" (which literally arranges safe activities into "light fare," entrees, and desserts — a primer in seduction that mixes and matches safe practices) does not distinguish between "homo" and "hetero" sexualities. It explains how to use both condoms and dental dams, the latter a device soon to be relegated to lesbian sex. Nevertheless, publisher Stephen M. Mindich and editor Richard M. Gaines are aware of the potential controversy provoked by the direct style, and the confusion that heterosex-

ual readers might experience in their first explicit exposure to practices they had probably assumed did not apply to them. Constructing their readers as a particularly sophisticated community, Mindich and Gaines suggest that readers can accept explicit information: "Because *Phoenix* readers are among the most highly educated and active people in our community — sexually as well as otherwise — the information presented in this guide has been written in a direct, candid, and technically conscientious manner" (p. 8). Nevertheless, the slight gap opened up by such phrasing between the publisher/editor and the reader/community also opens up the possibility of some readers deciding the AIDS coverage is for the benefit of other readers: "We value our readers and take very seriously our responsibility to do the best job we can in covering the major issues affecting their lives; there are few, if any, more important than AIDS" (p. 8).

(*Opposite*) This 1988 cover of *The First Against AIDS* by the Swedish National Commission of AIDS picks up a theme that reflected attempts by health educators to capitalize on the increasingly bleak virological news that the vaccine, promised by scientists upon the discov-

ery of the virus, was not at hand. At-
tempting to shift thinking from stopgap
measures awaiting a scientific break-
through to long-term behavioral and social solution, the magazine pictures a
thoughtful, tolerant, older woman who,
quite incidental to the overall message
of the spare cover, is herself Sweden's
Minister of Health and Social Affairs.
Her editorial (p. 2) reveals the complex
set of promises and threats that the
information-as-vaccine concept affords.
This is the logic that was soon developed into the national pedagogy in other
European countries and the United
States. Note how subtly persuasion and
confinement are juxtaposed, and how
the reader is presumed to be an unin-
fected person who might wrongly believe that discrimination will provide
protection from AIDS.

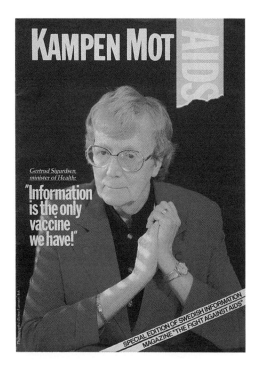

"... We know it will never be possible to completely control a virus that is
sexually transmitted. The infection has
found its way into our society, and it
will remain there for a long, long time.

"One way to [deal with this] is to institute new restrictions in society, and
increase the isolation of victims through
various controls. . . . Another way is
using information and influencing attitudes so that a gentler society is pre-
served. A society where it is clear that
HIV/AIDS victims have the same rights
as all other people. . . . Discrimination

must be prevented so that victims are
not afraid to discuss their infection; so
that they don't decline to be tested by a
doctor. Discrimination doesn't help halt
transmission of the virus" (p. 2).

But platitudes about human rights
and information provide the logic for
measures that do not seem terribly
"gentle." Sweden had already extended
existing STD control laws to cover people with HIV, making it a legal requirement for those who believe they might
have been exposed to HIV to seek testing. Each positive person was required
to discuss a "plan" for not transmitting
the virus to others and, if their supervis-

ing physician was not satisfied by the discussion, the person could be detained, as were several prostitutes during the time of the International Conference on AIDS.

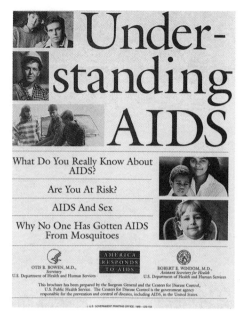

(*Above*) The 1988 cover of the controversial Surgeon General's Report fails to represent adult homosexuals, both the major object of discriminatory behavior and the group with the highest rate of HIV infection. Apparently, they were not among those with lingering questions about mosquitoes or risk.

(Opposite) Safer Sex Comix #5, "Leatherman," is one of the infamous cartoon booklets produced by Gay Men's Health Crisis in New York City. The booklets were culturally sensitive; they were sexually explicit; they demonstrated means to satisfying sex without taking any fluids into the body. By

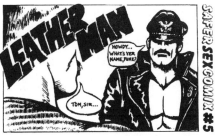
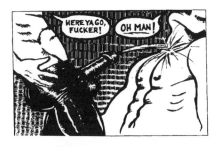
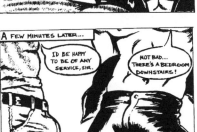
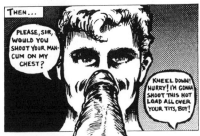
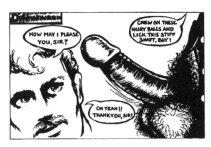
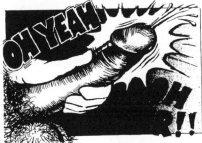
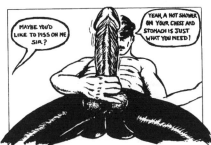
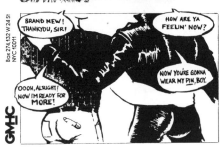

the end of 1986, it was illegal to produce them using government funds.
(Courtesy of Gay Men's Health Crisis)

(*Right*) This 1984 pamphlet, which I coauthored with Bob Andrews and Michael Bronski, is an early attempt to "eroticize" safe sex. Note that the term safe sex was not completely established. The pamphlet was designed to remind men vacationing in the Boston area (and especially in Provincetown) that they should maintain their preventive practices even while away from the familiar setting of their hometown. We avoided the usual format and worked out prevention logics through stories that mimicked pornography. We conceded to the perception that men still lacked basic information by including an explanation of the reasons why specific behaviors were known or believed to have a high or low association with sexual transmission of disease. The pamphlet, along with the Berkowitz and Callen (1983) booklet that helped frame it, was rare in adding some political critique: "The problem is we are treated as if we are too stupid to understand the medical information and too-sex-and-drug-crazed to evaluate our options. So, *they* give us lists of do's and don'ts. We've been getting this kind of sex education for so long that it makes us want to go out and do exactly what they tell us not to. With a vengeance [*sic*]. To make matters worse, after we've spent years figuring out an entire, ever expanding hanky code of fun things to do, now we hear

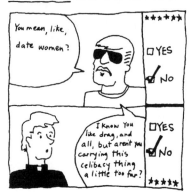

Sensible Summer Sex

You've spent that last six weeks at Tan-o-Rama so you won't look like a lobster after your first day on the beach. You've been doing double workouts at your gym. You and your travel agent have been through every possible hotel/plane combination to find *the perfect* vacation. You have thumbed through *GQ* on the sly to find out what you are supposed to be wearing and you've even bought the gay newspapers from the locale you are visiting, just in case there are in words or out places that you haven't learned of yet. But here's something you may not know: this summer's *hot* sex is *sensible* sex.

Wait. I know what you're thinking. You're going to toss me in the garbage. This isn't a lecture on body fluids or which positions you can't use *this* week. But if you want to have a really great summer — a hot, wild and sensible summer — you have a little preparation to do. So, here's some helpful hints from guys like you on ways they've found to have fun and stay healthy, too.

about 'safe sex.' It *sounds* like we have to give up all the excitement and become goody-two-shoes or wimps. But sensible sex can be just as hot and twice as healthy as your old bag of tricks. So grab your 'play safe' hanky (a black and white checked hanky popular at the time) and your 'ON ME, NOT IN ME' button. . . . Know the limits. Keep them. And then be as wild as you want. We are all we've got, so let's give this summer's hot sensible sex the very best shot we've got" (p. 2).

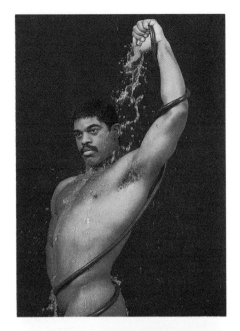

(*Right/top*) Graphic from a late 1980s version of "Hot, Horny and Healthy!" designed specifically for black gay men. The program was sponsored by the National Task Force on AIDS Prevention of the National Association of Black and White Men Together, and designed by members of the Los Angeles local chapter.

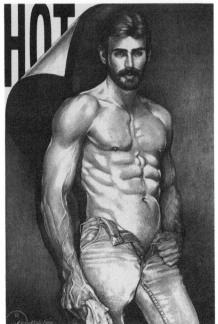

(*Right/bottom*) Al Parker generously offered us use of this image for the invitation to AIDS Action Committee's kick-off luncheon and press conference for Safe Company (1989). The image also appeared as a poster announcing the new peer education project in bars and other local gay businesses.

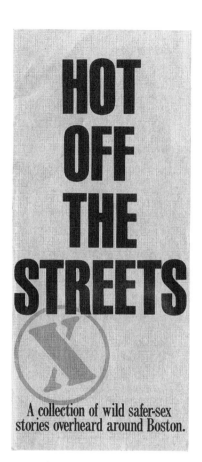

HOT OFF THE STREETS

A collection of wild safer-sex stories overheard around Boston.

"Hot Off the Streets" was conceived by the original steering committee of Safe Company and authored by an ad writer who volunteered with the group. Notice the anti-Helms disclaimer: "Funding for this brochure was provided in part by the Grass Roots Gay Rights Fund." In addition, the group decided not to include any list of risk-graded sexual activities, rather only the reminder: "Don't cum in his ass. Don't let him cum in yours. *Use a condom every time you fuck.*"

We tried to produce the stories as "real" by claiming that "these stories may change your mind about safe sex. There are some real sexy guys in our community who are having incredibly good safer sex. Maybe you could learn a few new tricks from them. Here are some of the hottest stories we've heard." We then solicited more stories for future editions of "Hot Off the Streets," which were unrealized. However, a clever volunteer did hijack a voicemail box on which to read pornographic safe sex vignettes: "If you've had a safer-sex experience that can top these and would like to share it, we'd love to know about it."

4

"The Only Weapon We Have . . ."

The national pedagogy operated first through media reluctance to discuss safe sex and then through the implosion of meaning produced by information overload. For the citizen, the individual process of learning compassion was homologized to the story of the epidemic generally: panic, confusion, acceptance. Even the impolite treatment/policy activism of ACT UP was an object lesson in the national pedagogy; activists' anger, especially that of people living with HIV or AIDS, stood in counterpoint to the compassion of the citizen. National pedagogy and safe sex education were reciprocal, in part negotiated through public health education programming and the evolving structure of gay communities, and in part contingent on an oppositional stance to each other. Safe sex could be mentioned but not explained: the bad sex that was the occasion for transmission could be described ("unprotected intercourse"), but the good sex that might end the epidemic had to remain obscure. Only militant safe sex organizing, officially declared obscene, remained outside the realm of citizen-like activity.

Even before the term "safe sex" was coined, gay men had begun to organize to avoid "acquiring" the hazily understood new disease. This early work, some five years before ACT UP's first actions, haphazardly fused the sexual politics of gay activists with the traditional health education models familiar to gay health care providers. This awkward mix formed the basis of an alternative safe sex pedagogy that, because of its nuanced and detailed understanding of sexual practice, could speak of sex in a way that made sense to gay men, while at the same time helping epidemiologists to investigate the specific modes of transmission. In this chapter I want to trace the development of safe sex organizing as a form of activism that challenged, but was tacitly incorporated into and reframed by, the official public health practices described in chapter 1.

Uneasy Convergences: "Safe Sex" from 1981 to 1986

The first safe sex projects were conceptualized during a period of extreme scientific uncertainty and broad fear of casual contagion. Early AIDS activists had to fight the callous treatment of people associated with the syndrome, while researchers and clinicians, who did not agree among themselves about the general progression of the new syndrome or its cause, fought about science. Some believed that there must be an etiologic agent that was most likely sexually transmissible. However, many others viewed the cause to be the "gay lifestyle"; use of drugs, perhaps even autoimmune response to semen, both were blamed for the observed immune system failure. In the context of this dissensus, "advice" developed by activists had to cover a lot of ground.

This was an excruciating time for early organizers: the number of men with "prodromal" symptoms who were projected to progress to AIDS increased almost weekly, from 5 percent to 10 percent to 100 percent, even as the projected life span from diagnosis got longer. In the face of extreme uncertainty, activists knew they needed to promote immune system protection and probably transmission disruption. But they also understood that they needed to work with scientists to gain insight into the syndrome's "natural history" and routes of transmission (if an agent *was* the cause).

Activist strategies evolved in relation to scientific developments. At first, gay men had to push to get epidemiologic studies undertaken, then they had to fight to ensure that research subjects still received safe sex information. Researchers ultimately complied, but the value placed on scientific study threatened safe sex education at every turn. Discovery of a virus and announcements that a cure and especially a vaccine were imminent sent prevention workers and researchers stepping on each other's toes: activists renewed efforts to sustain safe sex vigilance while researchers hoped to find "recalcitrant" people whose defiance of safe sex advice would make them good subjects on whom to test a vaccine. Scientists touted data showing decreases in new infections, but there were also concerns that safe sex education made vaccine trials problematic.[1]

Scientists hoped to solve the epidemic through biomedical means, viewing behavioral change as haphazard and impermanent. Activists sought immediate, gay community–controlled behavior change, viewing biomedical intervention as too late for those already infected and too uncertain for those whose infection could be prevented *now*. Scientists hoped biomedical intervention would reduce the harm caused by the virus after infection; activist educators hoped behavioral intervention would prevent transmission in the first place. Scientists argued that condoms were not "100 percent" effective, and that the use of any safe sex techniques was contingent on unpredictable humans. Activists argued that science was too uncertain: if sex was now conceived as a game of "Russian roulette," a vaccine or cure placed the pistol of risk in the hands of scientists who still did not understand the virus they hoped to conquer.

It was not until about 1986, well after the discovery of the virus, that the various ideas about risk reduction were consolidated under the name "safe sex," or later, "safer sex." It is hard now to imagine what it was like to organize for risk reduction with no single covering term; the title of the Callen-Berkowitz (1983) manual, "How to Have Sex in an Epidemic," recalls that time. But while it was born in opposition to a flat-footed homophobia that saw AIDS as punishment, the idea of safe sex failed to overcome the idea that queer sex was intrinsically dangerous. Once Americans were divided into citizens and deviants, safe sex became both required of and the mark of queers: queer sex had to be *made* safe while heterosexual sex *was* safe until queered.

From 1981 to 1986, there was virtually no official public sector education directed at gay men. From 1986 to the present, education efforts for and by gay men have faced extreme limits due to the Helms Amendment and the right-wing activism it has seemed to legitimate. But the limitations on safe sex education were not caused by direct censorship alone: both the Helms Amendment and the traditional health education theories that underwrote much early prevention work shared the premise that homosexuality could be neatly defined, and that the body who possessed it could be easily flushed out. Both assumed that homosexuals uniformly experienced and recognized — or could be educated to recognize — their condition. The early educational efforts from within gay communities, though explicitly opposed to the homophobically intended version of this proposition, came close to positing that sexual activities *are* equivalent to social identity, or at any rate, that practioners of same sex acts could be mobilized to a liberatory gay identity. Although they held radically different values about homosexuality, the public health system, the right wing, and gay activists all presumed a link between practice and identity and left it to someone else — health educators, clergy, gay liberationists — to posit the meaning of the homosexually performing body's activity.

Although conflicting and contentious, safe sex campaigns within gay communities probably helped ensure that individuals avoided HIV transmission. But in the long run, they failed to challenge the problematic split between "normal" and "deviant" sex, bringing the latter more explicitly under the long arm of the state. Gay men's and sex workers' sexualities and sexual vernacular were soon barely separable from the descriptions of them by state epidemiology. Programs varied in gay-positiveness and in their capacity to enable resistance to the social oppression that contributed to the failure to take up "safe sex." Most projects targeted individual competence and left unchallenged the social and political climate that influenced individuals' understanding of their sexuality.

Gay men's activist educational and organizing projects simultaneously questioned and relied on dominant concepts of behavior and sexuality. The trend toward incorporating safe sex into gay identity was both a resistance to and an attempt to be included in the emerging concept of the compassionate citizen. On one hand, reports about leveling seroconversion rates suggested that gay men could "control" their behavior: they were just like heterosexual citizens except in the gender of their object choice. On the other hand, safe sex organizers recognized that simple identification with the citizen produced disidentification with the safe sex advice that could prove lifesaving. Quite simply, the price of admission to the citizenry would be a disavowal of the relevance of safe sex, and, ultimately, the substantial spread of HIV among young gay men.

The phases of safe sex organizing I will discuss here were initially specific to a particular configuration of scientific knowledge, popular perceptions, and national efforts to describe the epidemic for the public: similar efforts today might hold quite different meanings and results. The early stages were marked by truncated information and a perception that scientists would quickly understand the cause and dynamics of the epidemic: any need for individual behavior change was short-term. By the late 1980s, however, there was a disabling information implosion that extended scientific expertise while making the simple meaning of information unreal to the individual who sought answers about his or her own means of avoiding risk of infection. The more science knew about AIDS, the less anyone seemed to understand about safe sex.

Speaking out about AIDS: Information Campaigns, 1981 to 1983

With some notable exceptions, the first risk-reduction efforts within U.S. gay communities, from 1981 to 1983, used straightforward information to identify and change the sexual and drug-use behaviors believed to be related to AIDS.[2] Inaugurated during a sense of emergency, scientific confusion, and a perceived media "blackout," these efforts almost necessarily began as "get the facts" campaigns that assumed that the major problem, or at least the first problem, was lack of information.

By degrees, the gay press became extensively and increasingly involved in alerting gay men about AIDS. When the epidemic began, there were only a handful of nationally and internationally circulated gay magazines or newsletters; however, most major cities had at least bar-oriented newspapers, and national and local organizations had newsletters that were used to get the word out. But while the early campaigns and the interventions of the gay press informed gay people internationally, both of the emerging health problem and of the backlash that accompanied it, there was little sense in the early years that the epidemic would actually spread across the globe. However, dispersion of information in the early gay press coverage and through organizational and friendship networks engendered a tremendous sense of mutual aid.[3]

The early gay media stories, and the pamphleteering and outreach efforts in the major cities, were vital in aiding activists to develop facility with once unintelligible scientific languages and crucial to individuals who were subjected to confusing, often experimental, clinical procedures. But in the context of a perceived media blackout, the information model that the gay media employed bifurcated knowledge into scientific and socio-sexual. Scientific knowledge was understood to be tightly held by the research and clinical system: activists should invade these systems to wrestle control over this knowledge, which was viewed as largely neutral in and of itself. Learning to talk science was likened to learning a foreign language; over time, words like retrovirus, T-cell, and immune suppression became (gay) household words.

By contrast, information about prevention was viewed as intrinsically political; any advice that was unwanted could be accused of being homophobic propaganda. For the most part, however, even the gay press viewed gay men as sex education neophytes. Early prevention campaigns failed to recognize that gay men were already experts on the language used to describe and enact sexual practice. If science information lost some precision in the hands of activists, then the campaigns of "don't's" (or "don't until") developed by clinics and health advocacy groups within gay communities lost sight of the complexity of sexuality. When the national pedagogy finally took off, gay activists found that the science information was too simplistic and the prevention advice too extreme. Gay media and prevention activists tried to produce scientific information that was ever more precise and safe sex information that was ever more user-proof and nonideological.

While the gay press and activist groups were lauded for bringing science to the people, early prevention campaigns came under fire from other gay people who viewed *themselves* as the true activists, sometimes even opposing gay groups they believed were too close to the official voices of sexual repression. For some U.S. activists, advice against anal intercourse was intrinsically homophobic. However, activists internationally disagreed about whether condoms were safe enough. Some Dutch and Scandinavian gay activists advocated abandoning penis-in-vagina-or-anus modes of penetrative pleasure, an idea considered ludicrous by heterosexuals and greeted as alarmist by gay activists in some European and all Anglo-American countries. Uncertainty about how long it might take to control the epidemic through medical intervention strongly affected activists' strategy: the optimistic viewed precautions as a stopgap measure until science gained control over the virus, while long-time gay health activists, who had faced similar promises concerning hepatitis B and other less fatal STDs, believed that change would and should be for the long haul.

Participation in the design of epidemiologic studies intended to describe sexual activity made prevention activists even more acutely aware of the gap between statistical concepts — "number of partners" — and the perjorative terms — "promiscuity" — that purported to translate data into individual advice. Linking the advice to decrease partners with a connotatively negative term put forward the worst interpretation of gay male sexual organization, overemphasizing total reported partners while misunderstanding the nature and quality of gay male social and sexual interactions. Some critics even opposed the advice to decrease partners, attacking both the statistics on which such advice was based and the misguided individual logic of "choosing carefully" it set in motion. Reducing partners required people to make choices on a case-by-case basis; instead of adopting universal precautions, people would develop selection strategies based in stereotypical notions about who was dangerous. Other critics pointed out that beating the statistical odds of encountering a person living with HIV by decreasing the number of partners only worked if the pool of potential partners was itself low in seroprevalence. For example, reducing numbers did little to reduce statistical risk if seroprevalence was 50 or 60 or 80 percent, as reported in some tightly knit groups of urban gay men, among drug users, and among presumptively heterosexual men with hemophilia A who had received factor VIII before 1985. By contrast, critics of selection strategies argued rightly, adopting transmission-interrupting techniques was equally successful in high- and low-seroprevalence situations.

In crude terms, the information deficit model that underwrote these first efforts explained the unhealthy behavior, located in the individual, as an effect of "ignorance." The solution was information. The model assumed two cases: first, that among ordinary people, information would change attitudes and awareness, which would in turn induce a desire to change, which would eventually result in change. In the second case, there was a breakdown in this normal progression: the informed person either would show no desire to change or would be unsuccessful at making a desired change. These latter two categories of individuals were viewed as recalcitrant or compulsive, refusing to accept the consequences of their problematic behavior or unable to control the drive toward it.

In retrospect, the problems with the information model are clear, as is its role in relation to the emerging national pedagogy. A major problem was the self-perpetuating claim about knowledge: as long as information was seen as effective in itself, rather than only the most preliminary beginning, lack of behavior change suggested that not enough or the wrong information had been provided. Information campaigns begot information campaigns, and social scientific evaluation of them begot more research. The complexity of administering such a volume of information about information stabilized health education institutions, which then had financial and political commitments to sustaining information campaigns and their evaluation.[4] But worse, the proliferation of more detailed and caveated information produced the illusion that risk reduction was highly complex and technical, a matter of percentages and mysterious fluid properties rather than familiarity with a condom and willingness to explore pleasures beyond intercourse. Whereas most people once learned their sexual techniques from discussion with friends or in action with their partners, individuals now got the impression that they would need extensive, even professional, assistance in sorting through safe sex practices. Beginning and sustaining transmission-eliminating techniques is complicated by social patterns and cultural values, not by biology. Learners were putting their efforts into studying the wrong information. They were trying to beat the odds by acquiring expertise in epidemiology instead of using and adapting their existing knowledge of their own socio-sexual milieu.

Finally, the assumptions of the information model, now crystallized as health education institutions, set a limit on government and social responsibility for promoting sexual health. Because the information model assumed that most people would respond in the desired way upon being informed, those who failed to respond — the recalcitrant or compulsive — were declared "hard-to-reach." To the extent that people so designated happened to match up to already constructed demographic units implicitly considered expendable — African American and latin youth, sex workers, bisexual men — officials and compassionate citizens could rationalize punitive actions — detention or simply refusing to intervene further. Instead of accepting the limitations of information campaigns, they blamed individuals' failure to change on stereotypical traits associated with the group. Despite its value in raising awareness and opening up access to care and support systems, the traditional information model, by denying the role of community norms in producing behavior change, led directly to punitive actions against the very people that the model failed.

From Precautions to "Safe Sex"

A second phase of gay-community–controlled, activist education, from about 1983 to 1986, tried to stave off the despair and incredulity that the initial efforts had left in their wake. These new projects had to adapt to rapidly changing ideas about the epidemic: the identification of a virus, the resultant increase in media coverage of scientific developments, and the first extensive media coverage of U.S. sexual mores revealed in the panic surrounding "heterosexual AIDS."

For the first three years, epidemiologists, activists, and those concerned about their health had focused on the past: how did AIDS start? What historical strengths in our community can we draw on? Did *I* do anything dangerous in the late 1970s? The discovery of a virus created a future.

With a slow-acting virus identified and probable routes of transmission already hypothesized, demographers and epidemiologists developed computer models to simulate the progress of the epidemic. Despite much criticized problems with the way these models constructed sexual networks, the data presented at the small, new AIDS conferences (widely attended by early activists — not primarily to protest, but to infiltrate the central place where one acquired a degree in "AIDSology") suggested that the future for gay men looked bleak. The ensuing focus on a single virus narrowed discussion of prevention to the disruption of HIV transmission only, initially disregarding the possibility of additional transmissible cofactors and discounting the more general immune-system-enhancing "lifestyle" choices that would prove crucial in slowing the progression from infection to symptoms and improving the quality of life for those infected. Precautions could no longer be viewed as an interim set of measures until medicine put things right: educators coined the phrase "safe sex" to mark a new approach to gay male sexuality.

The virus also gave the media something to *talk* about. Loathe to discuss the love that dare not speak its name, news writers replaced veiled allusions to dangerous lifestyles with medical reporting on the race for a cure and vaccine. Many in the gay community had become experts in this cutting edge area of medical research; now the general public could learn about the emerging knowledge about retroviruses. Those outside the gay communities (including homosexuals) would now receive far more information than advice. This coverage would become at least as important as that in the gay media in etching the landscape in which gay men lived the epidemic.

The sudden outburst of media coverage suggested that HIV had already spread dramatically and would be around for decades. But despite the apocalyptic stories circulating among heterosexuals, public health officials and the newly vociferous media advocated no *overall* change in the citizen's sexual techniques. Only gay men's sex required a total revolution in form. In this context, safe sex was very quickly interpreted by the mainstream as what gay men had to do. With the tide of increasing moral conservatism, calls to sexual austerity quickly overran calls for heterosexuals to also take up condoms as a universal precaution: the "sexual revolution" was over.

Heterosexuals should just do what they were always supposed to do: remain chaste until marriage and monogamous thereafter. If they failed, they should "choose carefully" and then take the "AIDS test" to find out if their radar had been correct. But while key gay ghettos saw a leveling of new seroconversions among adult men in the mid- to late 1980s, it was unclear that "waiting" ("increasing age of onset of intercourse") or "faithfulness" (decreasing number of partners) among younger people in high-prevalence areas would do any good. The failure to promote condoms as a cultural norm meant that when young people had sex, they did it without condoms — "the real thing" was their reward for waiting or for being faithful (at least, on a serial basis). As detailed in chapter 2, HIV infections among young people in cities where HIV was well established skyrocketed in the late 1980s, a trend that continues unchecked at the present.

In this new context, and as the logic of information campaigns worked themselves out in the face of the reality that "knowledge is not enough," two kinds of projects emerged: twelve-step groups of "sexual compulsives"[5] and workshops to "eroticize safe sex" designed by activist health educators. Both approaches were enormously popular and held out the hope of leapfrogging over the malaise of boring sex and into the brave new world of *safe* sex.

Fatal Advice

However, both supposed that gay men had a psychological deficit that could be remedied through quasi-therapeutic group work. Subjected to information campaigns that suggested change was easy, individuals who were unable to accomplish the recommendations of these campaigns, especially the decrease in number of partners advocated early on, easily concluded that there was something wrong with them, that they were compulsive. Gay men struggled daily against a culture that believed them to be pathological: since risk for HIV was popularly equated with number of partners and with homosexuality generally, what gay men had once viewed as a healthy desire for sex was reinterpreted as a pathological desire for dangerous sex, regardless of whether individual acts might be considered "safe." Groups for self-identified sexual compulsives may have created a safe haven for discussing fears about sex; they may even have promoted individual changes that proved lifesaving. But because these groups distanced men from the larger community, now viewed as triply dangerous (in twelve-step terms, full of dangerous "people, places, and things"), they fragmented rather than intervened in the structure of norm maintenance.

The "Hot, Horny, and Healthy" workshop, designed by Michael Chernoff in New York City and used since the mid-1980s, was an important step away from the behaviorist solutions that proposed abstinence in place of sexual activities now labeled compulsive or fatal. These workshops were probably most helpful during the years when the majority of gay men had experienced one cultural norm but now sought to reorganize their sexuality in accordance with an unclear new one. The workshops helped men who had naturalized one configuration of desires and practices to reconstitute their sexuality through eroticizing "safe" practices in the context of perceived new values of mutual responsibility and "communication." Unlike twelve-step groups, in which men stopped having sex and rebuilt their sexuality from the ground up, "Hot, Horny, and Healthy" was oriented toward celebrating and promoting already safe practices in order to replace activities that involved the indicted "exchange of body fluids." To sexual compulsives promiscuity was a slippery slope to desperately unsafe sex, but number of partners was not the concern of the "Hot, Horny, and Healthy" approach. Men simply lacked the skills to communicate their desires for safe practices and to make such activities erotically satisfying.

While it remains one of the most significant and widely used educational models, "Hot, Horny, and Healthy" made several troubling assumptions. It used a developmental model that assumed that sexuality must be tamed through mature and rational limit-setting, describing the 1970s as a mythical time in which "anything went" and rewriting the highly codified and ritualistic gay male culture of that time as lacking in norms and moral values. Invoking homophobic oppression and the "infancy" of the 1970s gay liberation movement, the pre-AIDS years were viewed as an adolescence for the gay community and its sexual values. The gay community was not pathological, but it was tragic that HIV had hit when gay men as a group lacked the skills — verbal communication and "intimacy" — required under the new constraints of the epidemic. Thus, "Hot, Horny, and Healthy" groups used exercises such as listing names for the penis in order to increase men's comfort with talking about sex, and role plays of diverse situations in order to broaden the circumstances in which they might "negotiate" safe sex. But the emphasis on verbal skills misunderstood the role of gestural, spatial, and symbolic modes of shaping and changing situational norms. In this approach, safe sex was less a transmission-disrupting choreography of bodies than it was an interview and contract for specific techniques.

While components of these programs dealt with nonpenetrative sexual options, they ultimately situated penile-anal intercourse as the most important form of sex, even if only as that which was lost and must now be mourned. Licking, rubbing, watching, fantasizing — the very practices that were once considered fetishistically absorbing and gratifying, and still the safest practices from the standpoint of HIV transmission — were tacitly reduced to poor substitutes, foreplay, or occasions for discussing the safety of practices to be engaged in later. The assertion of penile-anal intercourse as especially identity-conveying marked a significant change from the late 1970s ethos of the major U.S. urban subculture, where sexual specificity (transgression, fetish) rather than intercourse per se was the source of oppositional gay identity. This cultural shift in what constituted "real" gay sex precariously and dangerously rearticulated gay male sexuality and defined gay identity in terms of the one act that must be modified. In a sense, the new social definition of gayness, as merely different in choosing intercourse with men rather than women, narrowed men's sexual identity by staking it — gay or straight — on the performance of the most transmission-enabling practice. Gay sex was not only heterosexualized, it was made fatal by definition: avoiding inter-course altogether made one *safe* but not really gay, not really heterosexual, not really a *man.*

Thus, safe sex implied a loss of transgressiveness. This eliminated a crit-ical component of desire for men who continued to view gay sex as intrin-sically transgressive of cultural or individual psychic norms. With its hetero-sexist and Victorian unconscious, the safe sex practices eroticized in "Hot, Horny, and Healthy" were now overdetermined: safe sex demarcated trans-gressive sex from mature sex. But despite its collaboration in problematic theories of sexual development, "Hot, Horny, and Healthy" was not as indi-vidualistic or as moralistic as twelve-step programs. And, since they empha-sized big groups (in the first years there were often four or five hundred attendees), "Hot, Horny, and Healthy" workshops felt like "community" and performed the ultimate need to gain wide *social* adherence to norms.

Saving Sex/Liberating Sexual Community

During roughly the same time period, two different community-based safe sex organizing models emerged, one based on Paulo Freire's Marxist literacy projects and one grounded in gay liberation, itself a quixotic mix of 1960s new left Marxism, feminism, and the minoritizing discourse of the civil rights movement. The once widely used Stop AIDS Project, developed in San Fran-cisco and Los Angeles, was the first significant, organized move away from individual- or group-work-oriented programs. In its initial form, Stop AIDS utilized Freire's radical pedagogy, which was based on a diffusion model that assumed that social change occurred because an organized cadre of well-informed and motivated individuals effected change through their interac-tions with a larger number of people. Once a critical mass had been reached, the project could end, and community change would continue on its course. In essence, a vanguard would temporarily direct and speed up cultural change. The program trained a core group who then made individual contacts with other men, who were encouraged to advocate for safe sex in their community and among men with whom they had sex. Meetings reinforced community solidarity, conveyed basic safe sex information, and asked men to commit to building their community through safe sex advocacy. Although these highly visible programs boasted large numbers of individual contacts, their analysis of sexuality and community misunderstood the need to create ongoing interventions.

Stop AIDS did not adequately assess how sexual norms and changes in sexual practice were established and maintained in specific urban gay communities. Stop AIDS stretched Freire's literacy projects too far: while reading skills may be acquired, possessed, and carried around, "sexual literacy" does not easily translate from space to space. "No" does not reliably mean "no," and practitioners vary in their enforcement of rules depending on their partner and their spatially and temporally specific erotic goals. In creating a separate space for reflecting on the hazards of sex, rather than transforming the places in which sex happens to ones supportive of the new "safe sex" norm, Stop AIDS in the California context turned out to be more like a twelve-step program than Freire's literacy programs. Stop AIDS was always envisioned as temporary, vanguard projects to stimulate, and ultimately revert to, natural community processes: Stop AIDS did not provide an ongoing organizational mechanism for evaluating how safe sex norms were evolving, nor did the projects directly challenge sexual norms at the actual locations where problematic sexual practices were thought to occur.

By the late 1980s, groups in several cities (Austin, Texas; Sydney, New South Wales; Boston, Massachusetts; ACT UP in a variety of locations) moved toward another form of community organizing, advocating for safe sex through projects grounded quite overtly in *gay* liberation and in social construction theory, rather than in false consciousness theory. These projects viewed the practice of sex to be highly site-specific and expected participants to differ widely in their identities and motivations. Seeking sex and seeking relationships were viewed as two different enterprises, often accomplished through different strategies and in different locations. Organizers had to work, and work differently, in a wide variety of venues with unique norms.

Like the Freirean literacy projects, a core group of participants began a critical exploration of the meaning and rules of their own specific sexual worlds. They made conscious the norms and problems they confronted and solved daily; safe sex was not a problem, but a norm in process. Positing that a culture that supports gay male sexuality would support evolving changes in behavior and norms, these projects promoted positive attitudes toward gay male sexuality generally. They included safe sex practice as part of what makes gay sexuality an important source of community: working to make sex safe was an act of resistance to a homophobic culture. Although achieving specific changes in behavioral norms was urgent and imperative, the larger goal was promoting community processes that increased the resilience of gay male culture as a whole. Safe sex was viewed as part of the larger and ongoing project of sexual liberation; organizing did not end when a specific behavior change had been accomplished. Instead of being a separate and individualistic campaign for personal change, safe sex organizing was to be closely allied with both HIV/AIDS support and gay liberation projects.

This latter, emancipatory model challenged three features present in virtually all other forms of safe sex education: the understanding of safe sex as a stopgap measure, the premise that gay communities were chaotic and normless, and the description of the 1970s as "then" and the 1980s as "now." Instead, these projects celebrated the continuity and usefulness of sexual styles and negotiation patterns from the 1970s and 1980s.

The stopgap view of safe sex was seen as problematic for several reasons. First, it proposed the wrong motive and strategy for change — something like giving up certain foods until a weight-loss goal is reached, with no plan for addressing the personal or social factors that would need to be changed if the goal level is to be sustained. The interest in and even naming of "relapse" was a product of the stopgap premise: "relapse" blamed the individual instead of asking why a local culture failed to support the lower-risk activity. Second, the stopgap approach was grounded in scare tactics and explained an individual's lack of change as fatalism or compulsiveness. Finally, the stopgap view explained the social backlash dramatically accompanying AIDS as AIDS-phobia, rooted in ignorance, rather than as rewritten forms of basic and persistent homophobia. The reported increases in queer bashing and the expansion of more diffuse negative stereotyping were caused by individuals' ignorance about and fear of AIDS, not part of a larger and continuous system that discriminated against gay people.

Emancipatory projects also argued that the perception of 1970s gay culture as chaotic and normless was self-defeating because it was incorrectly based on the premise that sex was a drive that tended toward specific goals that had now to be diverted. Instead, these projects viewed sexuality as constantly in the process of construction and resymbolization. Thus, the gay identity associated with expanding sexual opportunities could be transformed into one that viewed safe sex practices as liberatory extensions rather than "mature" limitations. These projects assumed that preepidemic gay male culture had been highly organized with strong and easily understood norms that supported both the formation of community and the production of individual gay identities. The sheer volume of books, travel guides, and folklore — from jokes to hanky codes — about how and where to pick up men belied the inarticulateness of 1970s gay norms postulated by early programs. The norms of the 1970s may not have been recognizable as "communication," and were frequently not "intimate," but the semiotic codes and venue specificities were reliable; an individual could follow the migrations and changes in style employed by gay men to avoid policing and easily find types of sex or styles of men at particular bars or in particular places. Community norms had become so well integrated that they were no longer consciously perceived as constraints or requirements.

These projects also rejected the idea that the exigencies of a health "emergency" required a radical break from the sexual ideology of the recent past. They opposed moves to vilify or idealize the 1970s as a time of individual sexual license and community adolescence that needed to be replaced by individual and group maturity. Gay men's collective history — including an affirmative view of the 1970s — formed a basis for, not an impediment to, new norms called "safe sex." The emancipatory projects took pains to incorporate these memories of resistance and to celebrate the recent gay past. They assumed that community norms changed more quickly when men identified old rules as a positive process to be adapted rather than perceiving themselves to be isolated individuals moving from an unrestricted culture into one now rife with rules that must be learned as a novice.

The key insight of these community organizing projects was the recognition of differing sexual agendas, even in the same place, even between two mutually engaged sexual actors. However, the overemphasis on the value of an identity that could claim the gay liberation memories of resistance tended to reify the idea that acquiring a positive gay identity was a prerequisite to practicing safe sex. While this may have been somewhat true, to the extent that individual men followed the well-worn paths of "coming out" into the major urban gay communities, emphasis on an identity that transcended time and space distracted attention away from the constitution of norms *in* space. For the Freireans and the gay liberationists, norms adhered in the minds of individuals who collectively comprised the normative structure. The symbolic geography of particular spaces — and homosexual sexual culture broadly — was viewed as only occasionally having the capacity to hold norms in place. The shortcomings in the community organizing model became clear as activists transported this work abroad and tried to extend it to men whose identities were more contingent on class, race, or geography than on their sexual practices with men. Individual and collective change in sexual practices and norms is inevitably embedded in the larger national context, with its ambivalence about sexuality and its shifting fantasies about who comprises the citizenry that populates it.

Both Freireans and gay liberationists treated safe sex as a real thing instead of recognizing that "safe sex" is a transient ideologic construct forged in the desperate tension between the longing to be a citizen and the struggle to survive. By the end of the 1980s, safe sex was less a nominative category for a set of acts than a link to identifying with or rejecting the need to practice the technē that inhibit HIV transmission. Like the information model, both became sidetracked (even when producing pornographic projects) by specifying the menu of safe activities. They were overwhelmed by anxiety about giving accurate advice instead of recognizing that whether "safe sex" sticks is dependent less on its technical accuracy than by how transmission-disabling activities and their symbolic meanings are produced and reproduced within communities and spaces. Both recognized that changing same sex sexual norms requires strengthening communities, but this insight was dampened by their belated recognition of the hazards of an overly narrow concept of sexual community. Since many, perhaps even most, practitioners of same sex relations do not identify with a community, especially one that calls itself "gay," it was crucial to also analyze situations. Those active in emancipatory projects have hotly debated the value of promoting gay identity, but there is still not a solid case for comprehensive, global promotion of the urban-core-type gay identity. The issue is, of course, complicated by the relative success in carving out safe spaces for homosexualities in liberal democracies — the political formation out of which contemporary U.S. gay politics emerges and on

"The Only Weapon We Have . . ."

which its globalization seems contingent. However, the move from identity and community to venues and forms of homosexual practice that I will propose in the concluding chapter offers new means of exploring the political possibilities of other forms of queer activity while still making sex safe, even for those who do not accept educators' offers of identity and attachment.

Extending Safe Sex: Culture and Voyeurism

By the mid-1980s, it was clear that the materials produced within and for the core of the gay community did not hold the same meanings for white men on the periphery of gay life, much less for men with articulated racial, ethnic, and class identities. Groups "adapted" existing programs and began to "reach out" to these other gay men: the Centers for Disease Control even funded a project to adapt the "Hot, Horny, and Healthy" workshop for gay men of color, but there was a limit to the flexibility of these psychobabble, middle-class-oriented formats.

Often schooled in Rainbow Coalition politics, dissident safe sex organizers began to recognize the need for "culturally sensitive" and "sexually explicit" projects: government agencies also began to promote the former, even if they were still unwilling to fund the latter. But both terms were already overdetermined: culturally sensitive suggested a hands-off, community self-determination ethos, just what community organizers wanted. However, sexuality is not largely considered a culture in itself, rather, an artifact *of* cultures. Conflicts over *style* impeded efforts at cross-cultural coalition because ethnic or racially self-defined communities did not always share the feminist and gay liberationist impulses that had proved crucial to the early development of AIDS activism and safe sex organizing.

In fact, "cultural sensitivity" never really applied to sexuality within cultures. Programs designed under this banner rarely took account of the complex means by which heterosexism was reinforced as the "norm" in the culture toward which they expressed sensitivity. Culturally sensitive programs from ethnically and racially identified communities were not only often at odds with those coming from the gay communities, but, as feminists and queers of color pointed out, were overtly problematic for women and for the sexually nonnormative within those ethnic and racial communities. If white gay men often failed to understand the issues and experiences of people of color (including lesbians and gay men of color), it was some time before straight leaders from ethnic and racially identified communities were willing to acknowledge the sexual diversity in their ranks.

Cultural sensitivity, then, was often a cover for a sexual endo-colonialism; as effected in programs, cultural sensitivity ultimately came to mean the way *those* people who couldn't understand straightforward medical terms talked about sex. Outside the gay communities grappling (however badly) with their own diversity, cultural sensitivity became a new form of voyeurism for public health officials and clinicians who mastered the quaint vernacular of their charges. The discourse of gay activists and public health practices both measured the "need" for cultural sensitivity against a middle-class, white norm. "They" were more than simply different; lacking in both the decoding skills and the behavioral and social values of the mainstream society, "they" were deficient at best (gauged by whether they "changed" once they received the "culturally sensitive message") and potentially recalcitrant. The pedagogic practices that were deployed under the rhetoric of cultural sensitivity — tough talk pamphlets, "addict" educators — reinforced the idea that belatedly identified educational objects were unlikely to change. Instead of leveling the educational playing field, cultural sensitivity rationalized and perpetuated the bifurcation of target audiences into those who could be counted on to respond appropriately, and those who could be medically penalized and held legally liable for the lack of knowledge their risk behaviors were presumed to represent — whether or not they *actually* received education, sensitive or otherwise.

Cultural sensitivity was the opposite of the tendency to soften medical terms that might seem offensive to some groups, notably those not perceived to be "truly at risk." Though not described as *culturally* sensitive, educators were expected to tread lightly on the delicate sensibilities of mainstream heterosexuals whose privacy was to be respected at any cost: we were to talk of "making love" rather than the scientific penile-vaginal insertion or the bawdy fucking. In other groups, like gay men, cultural sensitivity meant not blinking an eye when speaking of rimming or fisting as opposed to anal-oral contact or manual-anal insertion. In all cases, cultural sensitivity required scientists begrudgingly to give up their stuffy clinical terms in order to water down the "real" and "specific" language for sex into derivative popular terms considered less accurate, but that subgroups of lay people could comprehend.

Despite the nod toward pluralism, the culturally sensitivist framework posited a reality of acts existing prior to the meanings created around them and constructed a double-entry system that equated acts with correspondent, technically correct words: folk terms were slightly confused translations. The task of the culturally sensitive educator was to match up existing folk terms with their corresponding scientific terms in order to ensure that the message conveyed was unhampered by its articulation in the less valued language. The process involved treating folk concepts as found and static artifacts of a pre- or protoscientific thought system: the educator was "sensitive" when he or she left such language as it was, while covertly determining its match to the proper terms.

Culturally sensitive educators ignored the ways that they policed sexuality through this enforced system of linguistic equivalencies. Polysemous folk terms that once enriched, altered, or reinvested local, sexual symbolics were reduced to one meaning once they were forcibly and publicly entered into the dominant discourse. Even the term fucking — once a term with a wide range of connotations — became the unified term for penile-anal or penile-vaginal intercourse, that is, for the potentially "bad" thing. Culturally sensitive educators also ignored the polysemy of clinical language; what, exactly, is a body fluid? Is "sex with multiple partners" an orgy or a parade? Uncritical cultural sensitivist educators and clinicians presumed the self-evidence of their own science language and made it the standard for accuracy. They celebrated the richness of the indigene's speech, but this aesthetic appreciation masked their inability to understand the fluid meaning of folk terms; irony, ambiguity, and double entendre were simply surpluses in their scientific system of equivalencies.

Although educational talk happened in the folk language, some amount of cultural violence occurred when terms were ripped loose from their practical contexts. Folk terms reappeared on charts and graphs at scientific conferences, where they were used to shore up the lack of reliability in quantitative measurements of sex with the illusion of qualitative intersubjective validity. Educators used folk terms in pamphlets and posters, hoping they could decrease the distance between themselves and those into whose lives they hoped to intervene. But these appropriations flattened out the folk terms, which lost their suppleness and the specificity that had given them moral force when used in the proper place and time. References to jimmy caps in rap songs wonderfully celebrated the adolescent penis and made the condom seem like a crucial fashion complement. But when used in safe sex pamphlets, jimmy caps rang false. However proficient the accent, folk terms were never quite used appropriately when pronounced back into the culture from which they had been hijacked.

But it wasn't just sexual deviants who objected to the scientific appropriation of folk terms for sex. Interviewers for the pilot study for Britain's national sex survey (Welling 1989) encountered extensive, if unorganized, popular resistance to the mislocation of sexual vernacular. Even though they often did not fully understand or recognize the terms, people preferred interviewers to address them in medical-sounding language. They were embarassed to admit to knowledge of terms that they used only during sex. Well into the epidemic, these respondents may have felt compelled to pretend to "accurate" knowledge by using (even incorrectly) words that sounded like those scientists would use. Likewise, injecting drug users and street teens felt offended or invaded when outsiders used their vernacular; they sensed that the professional was using the street terms "in quotes," policing rather than truly helping them.

Linguistic Orientalism

The idea of sexual explicitness also bore a realist mark, as if somewhere there existed a bare, mirror representation or language of sex. But instead of filtering "correct terms" through a posited "culture," the sexual explicitist framework viewed the downest, dirtiest words as most accurate to the user: anything less than unvarnished prose was a mark of repression. Linguistic transgression signaled a sublime realism, an erotic ground zero that kept escaping speech. Bawdy terms placed sex in a corporeal rather than a clinical context. But when used in clinical discourse, bawdy terms were treated like foreign words that have become standard usage but remain italicized to indicate their perpetual otherness and their magical power to *remain* untranslatable. But because bawdy terms were perceived by explicitist translators to have a privileged relationship to corporeal or sexual reality, there was no mechanism for deciding *which* bawdy terms to use, no assessment of the context or mode of address in which the terms were conveyed, no appreciation for the ways in which educators' use of these sexual rhetorics reinscribed systems of power.

Instead of investigating specific, local terms as they operated multiply and performatively in their contexts, educators operating from the most naive sexual explicitist framework used their own discomfort or amusement with "dirty words" as the criterion for closeness to sexual reality. This replaced straightforward sexual imperialism with an equally devastating romanticism based in the repressive hypothesis: dominant culture's rejection of "talking sex" in bawdy terms was taken as a *validation* of those terms. But when a subaltern group, unconsciously idealized as "naturally" less "uptight" about sexuality, rejected those very same terms, the explicitists viewed the subalterns as lacking in the verbal tools to express their unhegemonized sexuality. Incorporating, for example, gay terms into the grammar of the heteronormative discourse *shared* by dominant society and its clinicians might transform practices, but not because the combination provided better tools. Grafting reconstituted the subgroup in the terms of the larger culture; substituting "fucking" (a term favored by gay men over penile-anal intercourse), intercourse, or just plain "sex" (the term for penile-vaginal intercourse that seems to predominate in heterosexual circles), confounded risk reduction pedagogy. Stripping "dirty words" out of context and inserting them into another culture's linguistic system of sexual constructions obscured the ways in which those words police, constitute, resist, and protect sexual identities and subgroups.

Education by gay men, for gay men, was initially offered as a mode of breaking the silence about AIDS promoted by the nascent national pedagogy: the first break was information in any and all forms. As control over spreading the word shifted from a small number of well-informed and politically engaged groups to the mainstream news media, and as divisions in strategy arose among AIDS groups, safe sex advocates began seeking teacher- and learner-proof ways of communicating about safe sex. They shifted from organizing to *teaching,* from building a social movement to recuperating deviants in the national crisis over speech and its moral value. The nation could speak of gay sex not because there was an end to "denial" by the media or a national "waking up" to the seriousness of AIDS, but because the nation had embarked on a frantic attempt to regain control over producing heterosexual citizenry. Gay men rapidly achieved global publicity only to be overtaken by national pedagogy, whose idea of gay community was opposite of the renegade perverts whose very articulateness threatened to make deviant sexual arrangements appealing despite the presumed presence of HIV in those relations. The national pedagogy asserted that information should be neutral and value-free: it should not overtly blame gay men, but neither should it advocate homosexuality. Gay people continued to try and promote a particular (or several) interpretation of "safe sex," but "safe sex" slipped from a radical rallying concept to an apparently self-evident term rendered meaningless in the spiraling increase in information within the national public.

Most educators from within the hard-hit gay communities were convinced that explicit, sensitive materials representing sexual cultures as diverse as clones and sadomasochists were essential to changing sexual norms. However, most public health officials were convinced that bonding (by serostatus) and not bondage was the best means of halting transmission of HIV. The Meese Commission on pornography and the increased visibility of antiporn activists suggested that obscenity was dangerous, proliferating, and invading the nation: the fear that safe sex materials would leak into the mainstream and promote homosexuality doubled the fear that HIV was "leaking" out of its subcultural spaces. But militant educators only became more extreme, trying any means necessary to produce safe sex without reducing eroticism to information.

Finally, they went too far.

"The Only Weapon We Have . . ."

5

Visualizing
Safe Sex

Debates over who — government, communities, individuals — was responsible for safe sex raged on. Everyone from scientists to street hustlers quibbled over the details of what was safe, saf*er,* or safe enough. But educators were still faced with the problem of designing programs and materials that would help create environments in which men construed safe sex as positive, expected, and sexy. From the earliest years of the epidemic, radical educators and filmmakers toyed with the use of sexually explicit material. On the most basic level, teaching safe sex was a one-on-one affair, and many projects coyly proposed that men hit the streets to teach their brothers. Extending the idea of eroticizing safe sex, pamphlets and videos increasingly used second person address and imitated the style of gay male erotic literature. By the late 1980s, this kind of safe sex cultural work was in full swing. But their culturally specific erotics ran afoul of social attitudes: Jesse Helms gained support for a rider to the AIDS funding bill that prohibited promotion of homsexuality or promiscuity by raging against a series of sexually explicit pamphlets from the Gay Men's Health Crisis. Activist educators were already conflicted among themselves about how far to go in producing explicit materials. The potential for harassment by right-wing legislators added a new constraint on their ability to freely try out novel approaches.

Inevitably, educators turned to pornography, already a widely used popular art and a medium around which gay activists had mobilized before.[1]

Despite holding widely differing theories of the relationship between sexuality and textuality, porn producers, educators, and community activists were, by the mid-1980s, beginning to collaborate on safe sex projects. A range of questions ran through discussions about these projects: Is sex a drive, even a compulsion in some men? Could men make choices about safe sex? Did certain environments lessen one's ability to stick to safe sex? Could someone consent to unsafe sex? Whose responsibility was an individual occasion of unsafe sex? Who was responsible for establishing new norms? In 1989, I was confronted with these issues firsthand when, as a staff member at the AIDS Action Committee in Boston, I worked on an innovative safe sex project for gay men.

Signifying Safe Sex

Eight of us sat late into the night watching the same videotape again and again. We ran the tape forward and backward, ran in freeze-frame and in slow motion. The cleaning man finished up and hurried past us, obviously disgusted that four men and four women were staying late at the office to watch homosexual pornography. But sexual desire was not the source of our obsessive watching: we were searching for a condom. The actor had donned one early in the film, but once he began fucking, it was nowhere to be seen. We freeze-framed and scrutinized the base of his dick. We considered whether he might be wearing the new ultra-sheer condoms with no nubby end ring.

"Well, I don't see it . . ." said the videographer, a long-time Marxist lesbian activist.

"There! There!" exclaimed the design assistant, running back and forth through a short segment and jabbing his finger at the screen. "See that? It's shiny *here* and not shiny *there.*"

This was not a censorship board, although our discussions sometimes had a moralistic tone. No, we represented, in varying combinations, professional sex educators, academics and students, seasoned community organizers, professional filmmakers, and ordinary gay guys who wanted to make a contribution to slowing the HIV epidemic. We had come together, in 1989, to design and produce an innovative, multiphase safe sex education project by and for gay men. After months of reviewing other projects and discussing strategies, we decided that promoting safe sex in Boston depended on creating an environment in which gay men's sexuality was once again celebrated and in which safe sex was assumed to be a *norm* rather than a *problem*. Part of the project included intercutting a recent porn film with graphics introducing our project. But we encountered a problem in selecting segments for the trailer: how do you signify safe sex?

Was it that magic edge of the condom, the line between shiny and not-shiny? If condoms were obviously donned early in the film, would viewers assume their presence later, even if the condom was not obviously visible? Was "condom continuity" necessary — must we see the condom applied *and* removed in the technically proper manner? What did viewers make of the by then standard caution at the beginning of commercial porn tapes that all actors are practicing safe sex, but editing may have made this invisible? What about nonpenetrative (but still condomless) forms of safe sex? If adding a condom showed a change to safer sex, how could activities that required no change — like licking and jerking off — be resignified as still/already safe? Should porn simply show safe sex, or must some signifier of sexual danger demarcate the change in practices that were to be constituted as "safe sex"? Did all the heavy-handed efforts at eroticization implicitly suggest that safe sex was boring, thereby making unsafe sex seem even more erotic? Did eroticism arise more from the acts or from the narration, from the prohibitions or from the identities surrounding them?

By 1989, educators and commercial gay male video porn producers were converging on a new regime of sexual representation. Commercial producers wanted to be "responsible," and educators wanted to be "effective." But the approaches that emerged were contradictory and rested on widely divergent views of the role of fantasy and of textual mediation in sexuality. Even our little group had dramatically different ways of interrogating the possibilities and requirements of signifying safe sex.

Safe Company: A Radical Experiment

After several open meetings and weeks of recruitment in local gay papers (punning the Marine Corps ads, we said we were "looking for a few good men"), several educators[2] working under the auspices of the AIDS Action

Committee of Massachusetts assembled a core group of about twenty-five men and two women,[3] ranging in age from nineteen to forty-five, who were interested in being part of an innovative new endeavor. In addition to reviewing safe sex projects, the core group looked at theoretical work on sexuality, the history of gay liberation, and the development of AIDS activism.[4] The original group attended a weekend-long workshop and retreat, where we compared life histories by drawing huge collaborative murals of our "coming out" stories. Some participants told stories of illness and death among their friends and lovers, while others expressed amazement that they did not know anyone who was living with HIV. No one declared their serostatus, and many of the key group members said privately that they had decided not to take an HIV antibody test. One man's father had recently died of an AIDS-related illness, and his mother also occasionally participated in our activities. In short, our group came from a wide range of experiences. Members brought strong feelings and fears about their own possibilities for contracting HIV — or discovering they were already seropositive — and their own mortality if they did.

We discussed and debated views about safe sex and the needs of our local community. There was by no means consensus: individuals ranged from gay liberationists to radical fairies to twelve-step adherents ("sexual compulsives") to Helen Hay followers and "just guys." After the initial meetings, the members of this original group named themselves "Safe Company." Subsequent recruitment and training produced an affinity-group–like team who engaged in innovative and sometimes militant safe sex work in the many places where gay men cruised — bushes, bars, public toilets, porn cinemas — places familiar to the various members of Safe Company.

The name "Safe Company" was carefully chosen — participants wanted to avoid appearing to be an elite group who had special knowledge or moral superiority. The group put a lot of effort into uncovering and discussing their attitudes toward S/M, transvestism, gender and age issues. Although not always comfortable with men who were different than themselves, participants were concerned to make the group inclusive, open to different men and different ways of understanding sexuality. The name was intended to suggest that anyone could "be in safe company" by openly celebrating the importance and erotics of safe sex. Contextualizing safe sex on the company/community/group level, rather than the individual level, was intended to resituate sex from a private, personal danger to a fundamentally *social* project. Not only could safe sex be hot, but working toward community-wide adherence to safe sex could be an act of resistance to the destructive political, social, and psychological effects of the HIV epidemic.

This was an ambitious project in the cynical last summer of the 1980s. Safe sex campaigns and slogans were considered gauche, even if fears of sexual danger had produced a marked clampdown on public sexual expression. All of the major urban gay communities seemed to pass through a phase of sexual austerity in response to the exhausting political and social demands of the epidemic. Boston, as bitter local debates about public cruising, bathhouses, and the new monogamy indicated, lived up to its reputation as one of the more sexually conservative U.S. cities. By the end of the decade, New York and San Francisco had recovered their sexual adventuresomeness. In contrast, Boston's "phase" threatened to become permanent.

To make matters worse, the organization sponsoring Safe Company was widely perceived to be prudish and even antisex, and there were few organized countervailing "sex positive" forces. ACT UP Boston's occasional safe sex zaps were useful but did not congeal into an ongoing means of changing local norms. In order to signal the difference between this project and earlier individualistic or psychotherapeutically oriented programs, we invited porn producer and star Al Parker, a Boston boy made good, to join Safe Company for that year's (1989) Lesbian and Gay Pride Weekend. Al Parker was chosen for several reasons that suggest the direction of and conflicts within the practice of interventive representational politics.

Al Parker, who died in 1993, was, of course, a nationally known porn star, but more important, his style and age made him easy to identify with for the clone generation of gay men, the thirty-five to forty-five-year-old mustachioed and Izod-shirt-over-denim cohort who had, among gay men at that time, been most visibly devastated by AIDS. Al Parker was also raunchy enough to appeal to the leather and denim crowd, who had long been active in AIDS volunteer work, but had been publicly disenfranchised by the major AIDS groups or quietly marginalized by the (only just) mainstreamed gay and lesbian community who associated them with "dangerous" sexualities, especially S/M, itself erroneously linked to HIV transmission. Al Parker had already appeared in several safe sex campaigns on the West Coast and had been a vocal advocate for safe sex in the gay media and in a controversial appearance on the Donahue show. He was said to require absolute adherence to ultrasafe sex on his sets and had produced a commercial porn video short that was a hot primer on the use of condoms, surgical gloves, and plastic wrap.

Finally, there was a historical reason to work with Al Parker: as co-owner of the only fully gay-owned commercial gay porn studio, Surge Studios, his career as an actor, writer, director, and producer of sex films for gay men spanned and mirrored the gay liberation era. Like other gay sex films of the early 1970s, Parker's work (with Falcon Productions) had stylistic or content cues that signaled them as "gay." Of a piece with the experimental porn of the early 1970s, which hoped to cross over into art theaters, these films signaled their participation in a new sexual openness rather than marking themselves as evidence of a sordid secret. Although clearly designed to make their erotic incitations easy to decode, Parker's early work was aesthetically closer to Kenneth Anger's *Scorpio Rising* than to the glitzy, dequeered gay porn that emerged in the 1980s.

Al Parker's works of the 1980s were self-consciously, and often humorously, stereotyped fantasies of male-male sex. But unlike his commercial competitors, Parker's films made direct reference to the ethos, territory, and problems of urban gay life. The men of Surge Studios were more diverse than the hairless hunks of his competitors. Parker's erotics relied on action, the heat of sexual scenarios, not the fetishistic parade of beautiful male bodies. In the stylistically homogeneous 1980s porn market, the men in Al Parker's films were much more definitively *gay*. The sexual content of the film's was equally important to us. Like many gay films before the explosion of home video porn standardized the market,[5] Al Parker's films were less insistent that intercourse provide narrative closure: a range of sexual activities were proposed as objectives in themselves. The retention of "perverse," nonintercourse practices formed a bridge between pre-AIDS experimentalism and a new safe sex ethos that broadened the vision of what might constitute "sex" in the face of condom malaise.

Parker's charming perversity appealed to us as we considered how we might launch Safe Company. Gay male sexual practice of the late 1970s and early 1980s — at least in the urban cores where HIV would first become evident — had included a menu of activities, most of which held no possibility of HIV transmission. Unlike efforts to "eroticize" safe sex, Safe Company hoped to retrieve already and always safe activities like jerking off, licking, tit-play, verbal scenes, etc., not by proposing them as substitutes, but by returning them to their former status as core elements of queer erotic life. Because Al's films had always included a wider range of already safe sexual practices, and because they featured a variety of men, Safe Company believed these films would work well in a safe sex project with gay liberationist underpinnings. We hoped Al Parker and his videos would help promote the idea that safe sex is perverse and fun, not boring or limiting, integral to the dissidence, not the citizening, of the gay male community. Parker's presence would immediately signal Safe Company's intent to aggressively promote safe sex, rather than equivocally inspire fear.

The group moved forward, planning a benefit East Coast premiere of Parker's new *Better than Ever.* We used an original, sexy rendering of Parker's famous, jean-clad body as a promotional poster for the project and as an invitation to an inaugural press conference and reception, where Al Parker, his manager, and project participants answered questions from the gay and straight media and skeptical members of local gay political and service groups. In addition to granting us use of the rendering, answering questions, and signing autographs, Parker had kindly given us permission to edit any of his films — including the new one — into a video that would introduce the project on the omnipresent screens and monitors of local gay bars.

And that is when the trouble began, not because right-wing forces intervened — we had already strategized with Senator Kennedy's office and earmarked a special fund of community donations to pay for the project. The videographers came back to the group with a distressing claim: *Better than Ever* was "not safe."

Containing Safe Sex

Better than Ever contained the usual notice to the viewer that all actors were practicing safe sex, but for artistic reasons, barrier devices might not always be visible. The actors indeed donned condoms before the camera's eye, but condoms were not always visible thereafter. Although a wide range of "safe" activities occurred—use of dildos, use of "stubbies" for fellatio (short condoms that cover the head of the penis)—"safe sex" was not signaled as "different" within the narrative of the film.

Was that safe?

The theoretical issues we raised about representation and interpretation must have been quite similar to those questions debated late into the night at art schools. Like activist artists in other cities, we were working on an immediate, practical problem. By reshaping cultural artifacts to revitalize a community under siege, we hoped to shift sexual mores and reduce the ravages of a new disease. Theory and practice could not be separated: each argument about the nature of representation, the meaning of safe sex, and the modes through which community change might occur was grounded by death witnessed and community destruction survived. While the arguments outlined below and my own theorizing about sexual vernacular (chapter 6) and their relationship to sexual spaces seem abstract now, they represented the core issues in an ongoing struggle for community self-determination.

During these discussions, it became clear that "safe sex" was a constructed category, naturalized through reference to medical research on transmission, but deeply dependent on local interpretations. But the relation (or distinction) between fantasy sex and "actual" sex, and the capacity of sexual agents to rework the symbolic meaning of particular acts, were far from clear. We disputed the nature of porn watching: is it a sexual activity in itself (a "parasocial relationship," to use the clinical term) or an aid to the imagination, doing the work of fantasy production *for* the viewer? Do viewers take videos to be real? What do people *do* with videos? Do they imitate what they see? Does watching "unsafe sex" enable men to vicariously enjoy (or mourn) practices now ruled out of bounds? Do "unsafe videos" image, stabilize, or even produce a desire for a set of activities that ought to be erased from collective memory?

These questions prompted controversy, anger, and accusations of, on the one hand, denying the reality of an epidemic, but on the other, denying the demands of desire: of allowing unsafe sex to continue, or of promoting paranoia about sex altogether. The dozen or more people involved in some stage of our discussions about this phase of the project each had his or her own stories to tell about their relationship to pornography, including never having seen any before, their own experiences of both sexual pleasure and sexual danger, their own visions of what a "safe company" might look and feel like. Three basic, partially overlapping positions emerged in our discussions, although there were no doubt many additional ways to approach the issue of whether or how to use video pornography in safe sex projects:

1. Videos must show proper application, use, and removal of a condom, in order, and with episodic framing that leaves no doubt about the pragmatics of condom use. The viewer should be able to clearly see the condom on the dick at all times, including when the actors are fucking.

This argument assumed that some measure of direct modeling occurs in the viewing process and that learning about condom use requires real-time portrayal. The primary stamp of safe sex advocacy in a video would be information-giving, not eroticization. Porn is by nature fantasy, leaving out "boring" or logistically complicated aspects of sexual practice in order to maintain sexual tension and get the maximum amount of sex on screen. Although pornography might be able to give information, the specific requirements of safe sex representation would probably be at odds with pornographic conventions.

2. The now-standard disclaimers that tell viewers that actors are practicing safe sex but that editing may make condoms difficult to see are effective at promoting safe sex. Viewers simply imagine that the condom is in place or, at any rate, do not imagine or desire its *absence,* that is, *unsafe* sex. Porn is understood by viewers as fantasy, but producers do not do all of the "editing": viewers supply or ignore any number of details or elements.

This argument assumed that safe sex was an already accepted norm in gay male sexual practice, thus, extreme visual punctuation is not required. Safe sex is a symbolic concept for a range of practices, only one of which is condom use. An overemphasis on condom use, especially by signaling its difference from unstated practices, comes at the expense of failing to celebrate the many other already safe activities.

3. There are no specific requirements for representing safe sex, although avoiding reference to the idea that safe sex is now an important issue ("going on as if nothing has changed") is not acceptable.

This argument assumed that a range of textual elements — narrative, overt representations, dialogue, the instructions before or comments at the end of a tape — each cue the viewer to interpret the film in the context of safe sex. Viewers are assumed to be already actively interpreting porn texts in the larger context of their lives and sexual practices. This argument assumed that individuals have a wide range of reactions to pornography that are strongly influenced by intratextual characteristics, like stereotyping or narrative structure, and by their viewing context. Interpretation and enactment of safe sex depend on cultural attitudes, not on the presence or absence of specific representations. What porn tapes say about gay male sexuality and how porn relates to the social context of gay male culture are larger issues than the specifics of condom visibility. Porn videos are useful if they suggest positive attitudes about gay male sexuality because that helps create and sustain a social environment in which safe sex is practiced *because* it is viewed as a positive aspect of gay male sexuality. Thus, nuances in pornography's narratives about sexuality and about interrelationships between men can promote the confidence men need to enact safe sex and not feel limited by condom use.

In the end, the group could not decide what constituted a representation of "safe sex" in time to make the most provocative entrance for Safe Company. (The effort was revived by the group in 1992, resulting in an explicit music video production featuring the "Hat Sisters.") But the debates surrounding the retreat from educational porn are worth recounting because they point to the issues that have complicated strategies of using urban gay men's sexual languages to mediate safe sex.[6] The degree of difference in these understandings of the role and function of pornography suggested that the media was itself in flux. Certainly, concern about the epidemic was a major factor in changing both the industry's style and educators' willingness to go out on a limb. But changes in technology, especially the rise of home video, also dramatically changed the style and marketing of pornography. The safe sex porn projects of the 1980s, several of which I will discuss below, must be placed in the context of this larger and radically changing video market.

Changing Markets, New Pornographies

Consumers of the 1980s who casually perused their video store's new selection of pornography were probably surprised to discover that mainstream producers had capitaiized on the virtually universal ownership of VCRs and crafted a range of new styles of pornography. This new home-viewing market made possible a variety of subgenres and, in particular, a narrative form that appears to have been marketed to new, upscale consumers who did not identify with the stereotype of the sleazy, perverted dirty movie viewer. Visual codes were reworked, and production values improved. Even the erotics of viewing changed: the fear of getting caught attending a porn movie was gone. The vacillation between voyeurism and exhibitionism that pervaded the XXX cinema experience was radically altered. Old terrors were replaced by new ones: the glance of the store clerk; the anxious survey to see if ones' neighbors were in the store; the dance to avoid the child rummaging through the Disney videos on the shelf below; the double check to be certain that the living room curtains were closed; the sound checks to determine what passersby might hear.

Ordinary video stores made some attempt to keep their blue stock separate, but there was no longer a strong sense of illicitness about obtaining the videos. Some stores put pornography in a separate room that (supposedly) only those over eighteen could enter. Others kept box covers in a book that was available on request. Some simply placed the videos bookwise on a high shelf, sometimes covering them with opaque sliding doors. Thus, the context and erotics of choosing pornography diversified. As opposed to selecting a *film* from among the many forms of skin offered in a combat zone, video pornography viewers chose pornography over some other type of video. With the rise of cable and pay-per-view pornography channels, viewers could even see pornography with no effort or planning.

The structure of erotic experience was now enmeshed with rather than opposed to routine consumer activities and domestic rituals; a couch potato, do-me ethos replaced the nomadic activity that once characterized the XXX cinema. Engaging in or watching sex with and among members of a cinema audience was replaced with the coy invitation to mate or date, to come up and see a few videos. TV screens buzzed with a panoply of disjunct images, and the separation of domestic pleasures into special rooms broke down: people consumed pornography in the same space, on the same machines, where they had watched the news, their favorite TV series, or the Weather Channel only hours before. The genre that had once been banished to the big screens of decrepit theaters in scary neighborhoods, to be anxiously and secretly viewed by strangers (the sense of illicitness was part of the price of the ticket), became the most public but domesticated form of sexual representation.

By the mid-1980s, U.S. home video pornography producers had created a variety of products to appeal to increasingly diverse viewers: both the cinematic conventions and packaging suggested that videos were aimed at and semiotically coded for specific audiences. Film titles and the photos on box covers suggested the gender and sexual orientation of the presumed viewer — male/female/transperson, gay/straight/cross/bi- or transsexual — but viewers defied any strict equation of identity and a preference for seeing homo- or hetero-eroticism. Many lesbians seemed to like gay male porn (at least until more by-lesbian products became available) and many gay men liked bisexual offerings. But did they desire the bodies, the plots, or the idea that they could have something forbidden? If the more traditional "girlie" movies produced the female body as fetish, videos with a strong narrative structure may have made it possible for viewers to ignore the gender of characters with whom they chose to identify. Indeed, the debates about female spectatorship had already suggested that women were accustomed to performing various cross-gender gymnastics in order to take pleasure in films. In addition, gay men have a long history of identifying with the tough or glamorous women of Hollywood films of the 1940s and 1950s. The new lesbian and gay male viewers, schooled more in mainstream narrative than in the complex semiotics of pornography, may simply have done what they knew best: bent the gender of characters whose roles they liked.

The increasing participation of new consumers — lesbians, gay men, and women generally — and the decreasing costs of producing and marketing targeted products afforded new opportunities for "minority"-controlled productions and for segmented interpretation of mass market videos. Because the emerging formats relied heavily on televisual and Hollywood conventions, they were probably more readily understandable to novice viewers: this diversification in pornographic styles created an opportunity for safe sex educators. Although they all feature no-shot-barred cinematography, the specific examples of safe sex pornography to be discussed below utilize a range of the new formats.[7] Offering erotic pedagogies in different formats to consumers with varying familiarity with particular modes of representing sex was certain to produce wildly disjunct interpretations of whether what they saw was *safe*. The taxonomic scheme I outline here was developed in relation to the video offering likely to be found in the porn section of ordinary video stores (in places where this is the mode of distribution). Although people who obtain videos from specialty shops or magazines may be able to find products exactly matched to their own specific erotic interests, the widely obtainable videos often cross sexual tastes, or encourage viewers to "read in" differences in gender. Thus, while the bulk of the categories below have both "gay" and "straight" versions, specifically lesbian and gay videos make innovations that fall outside the general offerings. Thus, this general scheme is designed to foreground possible differences in the interpretive frame viewers might apply to a video text, and, hence, suggest what subgeneric differences might account for different interpretations of "safe sex" in pornography.

1. A significant number of videos, especially at stores with a small stock, are dubs of widely screened classics of the XXX cinema heyday of the 1970s, films like *The Devil in Miss Jones, The Opening of Misty Beethoven, Deep Throat,* and *Debbie Does Dallas.* These high-production-value films were originally produced during the brief period when pornography was considered (by the first presidential commission) to be relatively innocuous. Serious, experimental filmmakers hoped their sexually daring products would cross over to those art cinemas that showed the emerging European soft core pornography like the Emmanuelle films and more serious films like *Venus in Furs.* Although they rarely even refer to "gay" sex, they frequently have a "lesbian" sequence. Gay films like *LA Plays Itself* had similar, if more modest, ambitions and influenced the first generation of self-consciously "safe" pornography, most notably *Play Safely* discussed below. Pushing the envelope of social tolerance and viewers' expectations, these films introduced narrative into sex vignettes, a strategy that emerged again in the 1980s as videomakers tried to attract viewers who were unfamiliar with the antinarrative conventions of older pornographies. However, they differed from their 1980s cousins in presenting oral and anal sex as taboo. The bulk of the 1970s films dealt with disinhibiting characters from fear of oral sex, a plot that seemed more related to fears of *vagina dentate* than to the superficial proposition that women won't or don't know how to do it. Anal sex was not a major preoccupation in mainstream film pornography until the 1980s, and then it was an *alternative,* not a *problem.* The immortalizing of these "classics" on

video means that post-VCR boom viewers can see the products even if they cannot recapture the thrilling transgressiveness of the group viewing of them.

2. Display videos are essentially moving versions of mainstream, mass market print pornography, produced by and matching the visual conventions of the major magazines. These films rarely have plot, usually contain no identifiable sex acts, and often feature women alone. The women in *Playboy Bunny Aerobics* may rub their bodies, but as an enticement to the viewer, not as a source of pleasure for themselves. The viewer's gaze is not directed through a male character in the video, although he is the "partner" to the woman in the video.

3. In cabaret videos, sexual vignettes are staged as a show. They have little or no narrative continuity, and the sex is explicitly produced as a performance, with the viewer situated as a voyeur, sometimes a member of the audience represented in the video. Although there are relatively fewer videos of this type, several important political interventions of the 1980s were composed in this format, including Marilyn Chambers's *Behind the Green Door* and its quasi-feminist, safe sex sequel, *Behind the Green Door, Part Two,* and *Cafe Flesh,* a post-apocalyptic/post-AIDS video commentary on the new moralism of the 1980s: nuclear fallout has rendered only a tiny minority capable of experiencing sexual pleasure without becoming violently ill. These people — called sex-positives — are captured and forced to perform live sex acts before sex-negatives who struggle to enjoy without getting turned on. These videos suggested that there were many possible erotic attachments, but any person would be attracted to only one: they had "something for everyone," rather than suggesting that individuals might be interested in all of the scenarios.

4. Gender fetish videos are like peep shows: types of women, rather than a narrative, create the continuity of the video. The women have sex, sometimes alone or with each other, sometimes with a man; however, no narrative tension or sexual problematic is created. Types of women signify types of sexuality that are already assumed to imply particular sexual scenarios. Thus, the plot, if any, is pat; we know what will happen as soon as we identify the female stereotype that governs the video (usually evident from the box cover). Unlike the coding in the narrative videos, in which sexual aims, race, and class are part of the problem of desire, in these videos, race, class, and gender sign fetishes: the videos "supply" a perceived demand for fantasy material

Visualizing Safe Sex

about women who look (and sometimes act) a certain way. The videos make very little sense if the viewer cannot decode the signs of race, class — or beauty or ugliness or fatness or age — *as* fetishes. These include videos like *What Kind of Girls Do You Think We Are?, Black Beauties,* and dozens of titles with "tits" in them.

5. Narrative videos seem to dominate the offerings at ordinary video stores. With their high production values and allusions to recent Hollywood films and television series, these new, nonfetishist, nonvoyeuristic videos *represent* sex. Typical names are *Beverly Hills Cocks, Edward Penishands,* and both gay and heterosexual versions of *Big Guns.* Clearly, their contingent relation to Hollywood's sexual elisions provides an erotic and humorous critique of the mass media's role in invoking but never delivering sex.

It is important to observe that anal and oral sex are routinely practiced in these films with no suggestion that the acts are "taboo": both practices are simply part of the menu of sex presented in the videos. Significantly, while "ordinary intercourse" predominates, both oral and anal sex can culminate in a come shot, somewhat decentering penile-vaginal intercourse as an identity-marking practice.

These videos almost always have a story that runs through and frames all of the sexual encounters. They combine realistic visuals, presumed to be the representational preference of men, with the romantic narrative structure apparently preferred by women (Radway 1983; Modeleski 1984). In a sense, this new format feminized pornography by using romantic conventions associated with soap opera. In marked contrast to anything else on the market, there is almost no indication that what we are seeing is in any way kinky or taboo.

Although visually and narratively similar, earlier high-production-value pornography revolved substantially around the cultural stigmas and anxieties about oral sex. In contrast, the 1980s narrative videos are about the sexual problems intrinsic to various, often stereotyped social *relationships,* not about the problematics of particular sex *acts.* Types of sex are rarely presented as taboo in themselves, only as representationally taboo — what Hollywood or television is unwilling to show.

The narrative videos aimed at gay men and women — heterosexual and lesbian — also differed from the earlier "lesbo" segments in not showing a tabooed sexuality that can only be seen here, but in showing a normal sexuality that society has proscribed. The emphasis on narrative continuity and linear portrayals of mutual erotic delight normalized the text as text: the videos seem intent on *not* marking themselves as a space of privileged encounter with sexuality.

The combination of new audiences and the use of well-worn Hollywood and televisual conventions in narrative videos altered the interpretation of pornographies. Of course, only ethnographic work can fully describe evolving interpretive strategies, but examining texts affords some insight into what commercial pornmakers thought their new audiences wanted, and highlights the diversity of cinematic logics that confronted those who sought to produce or consume new kinds of sexual representations during the emergence of the AIDS epidemic. Both the new commercial work and that of countercultural producers sought to normalize the desires they represented. If older, illicit porn tried to invoke for (largely male) viewers the sense of getting away with something, the new videos suggested that viewers were finally getting to see their own desires portrayed "realistically." Voyeurism was replaced by mirroring, not so much as a new realism than as a flat surface on which multiple desires could be projected. We weren't seeing someone else doing something we shouldn't be seeing, but we were finally getting to see what we ourselves looked like when we were doing what (we liked to think) we normally did. Porn was not reenacted but mimicked, subverted; it was not a manual for perversion but a site of memory of the body defying convention. This is some of the appeal that new pornographies held for the dissident safe sex educators of the 1980s. Although later work would be more influenced by radical young videographers, the following selection of early efforts include pornography that adds safe sex twists, videos produced for screening in bars alongside music videos, and videos that were specifically marketed as educational pornography.

Safe Text: Some Variations

Play Safely, 1986, directed by David McCabe, Fantasy Productions,
    in consultation with educators. Commercially available.

Play Safely uses flashbacks to produce a before-and-after structure that depicts gay men coming to grips with changes in their sexual culture. The film's premise is that a "brush with reality" (the encounter of a character who eventually tests antibody negative with a "promiscuous" man who is rumored to have AIDS) enables the men to make positive and hot changes toward safe sex. Like much narrative porn, the plot line weaves together the stories of several characters, allowing producers to show more types of men having more types of sex, presumably allowing a wider range of viewers to "identify" with characters and issues in the video.

The plot progresses as one member of each couple anxiously articulates a specific concern about their risk of contracting HIV. Their partners respond with words of comfort and wisdom, proposing various strategies — monogamy, testing, avoiding people who "don't look well" — but always employing condoms as the best solution. The narrative format allows the director to use extensive, sometimes didactic dialogue; as the erotic tension builds, the characters spin out complex logics of safe sex decision making.

Play Safely also displays the practical aspects of safe sex in exhaustive, almost tiresome detail. The "difference" of *safe* sex — and "safe" porn — is reinforced through flashbacks of an earlier time, when characters were having unsafe sex. The flashbacks — virtually identical to less self-consciously "safe sex" porn on the market at the time — are as hot as the ensuing "safe" scenes. While these suggest that safe sex is as erotically charged as unsafe sex, the juxtaposition also teeters on the brink of its own realism: the viewer is asked to believe in the recounted dangers in order to appreciate the importance of taking up safe sex practices in the film's (and viewer's) present. Like much safe sex advice that rests on a "that was then, this is now" strategy, the film constantly invokes the erotic appeal of the very sexual activities it is trying to reimagine.

Interestingly, the video contains a rare coming-in-the-condom shot. (Another appears in the trailer to Al Parker's *Turbo Charge*.) From the standpoint of demonstrating condom use, there is no good reason not to remove the condom upon pulling out, as many gay men do in "real life." The film does not appear to be suggesting that men actually duplicate this activity; instead, it seems to rework the ideologic structure of porn's traditional come shot. If the condomless come shot was a metonym for what was happening "inside," out of view of the camera, then the coming-in-the-condom shot visualizes condom efficacy. The viewer is reassured that the condom actually will contain coming, even if we can't "really" observe this happening inside.

Top Man, 1988, written, produced, and directed by Scott Masters, Catalina
Video and Newport Video. Commercially available.

With its humor and its extremely high production values, *Top Man,* one of the
top-grossing porn films of its year, set a new standard for casually incorporating condom use without didactically foregrounding safe sex. The use of
condoms is not problematized: all scenes of fucking include both condom
application and clear "meat" shots (penis-in-anus) in which the line of the
condom is visible. Two segments of dialogue about condom use are incorporated into stereotyped scenarios of "teaching" another man how to have
homosexual sex. The implication is that teaching about queer sex includes
teaching the use of condoms: the film inculcates a sense of collective responsibility for ensuring condom use. In a final orgy scene, there are plenty of
condoms for everyone, and everyone uses them without hesitation. Condoms
are completely normalized, both as something you can give to someone who
is not initiated into gay sex and something men can freely use and ask for
within gay culture.

Turbo Charge (trailer), 1987, written and produced by Al Parker and Justin
Cade, Surge Studios. Presented as a public service announcement.
Commercially available.

The trailer to *Turbo Charge* shows Al Parker and Justin Cade using condoms,
surgical gloves for fingering, and plastic wrap for ass licking. Reference to
safe sex as such is not made until the end title, which encourages viewers to
have fun and engage in safe sex. The smooth acting and ease with which the
men employ safe sex techniques suggest that this is simply what men do. The
men snap the condoms in mock dick-torture, suggesting not only that condoms are ordinary, but that they are an improvement on the game. Split-
second repeat editing provides viewers with a clue to the problem points in
safe sex techniques: getting the plastic wrap out and smoothly covering the
ass and getting the condom rolled down past the receded foreskin are highlighted without interrupting the flow of the sex. The five-plus-minute clip is
didactic insofar as time and care are taken to present the major safe sex
techniques, but the techniques are taught in the course of a scenario that
shows the men having fun and attaining sexual pleasure.

Visualizing Safe Sex

The Gay Men's Health Crisis Safer Sex Shorts, 1989, directed by Gregg Bordowitz and Jean Carlomusto. Three to four minute shorts available from education outlets and some video stores.

These clips are part of an ongoing project by activist videomakers working with community groups to create vernacular safe sex representations. The first two were screened at the Fifth International Conference on AIDS in Montreal in June 1989: *Something Fierce* is a rock-video-style guide to fantasizing, touching, and fucking using a condom, including a didactic interlude in which the dancer applies and removes a condom from his own penis. *Midnight Snack* shows two men meeting at the refrigerator and using whipped cream and honey to sweeten fellatio (with a condom). Neither shows the traditional come shot, but both signify sexual pleasure through the men's facial expressions.

Car Service, designed by a black gay men's focus group, is organized by a more typical porn narrative: a yuppie black man discovers he has lost his wallet and pays his macho black cab driver with three condoms. The cab driver pulls into a quiet place, and the men have sex. Although we see the condoms, a penis, and a greedy, winking anus, we do not actually see the condom applied, the penis inserted, or a "meat shot," even though the men appear to have anal intercourse. The focus group preferred an erotic, soft core representation in which the condom signifies both anal sex and safe sex. The video is an implicit critique of the more hard core, fuck-focused eroticism of mainstream, largely white, gay-male-oriented porn.

Current Flow, one of the first projects in the world to promote safe sex for lesbians, acknowledges that the concepts, techniques, and tools of safe sex are new for most lesbians. One woman interrupts another who is masturbating and unrolls a towel containing the full complement of safe sex devices. The camera pans slowly over dental dams, surgical gloves, lubricant, and a dildo (a feminist, antirealist one that resembles a gourd more than a penis). The camera pan, which was commonly used in early gay male and heterosexual safe sex educational films, introduces a critical didactic element for the then new audience of lesbians concerned to learn about safe sex. The women engage in a variety of activities, employing all of the latex accoutrements. *Current Flow* is remarkable both as a safe sex video for lesbians and as an early contribution to the emerging field of lesbian-produced lesbian erotic film. The video sets itself apart from lesbian scenes in traditional, heterosexual-male-directed porn through its use of women's music in the background.

Clearly, the early efforts at creating pedagogically directed erotic films produced a range of results, some of which were marketable as "pornography," some of which seemed to stimulate dialogue about sexuality more than it served as a primer for or incitement to specific practices. In each case, the reworking of traditional genres to reflect new anxieties stressed the existing languages of sexuality. The various uses of identity, the disruption of desire, and the introduction of supposedly new techniques created hot new products for some people, but ruined the appeal of a long-loved genre for others. One result of the debates about these works was the recognition that the relationship between codes designed to negotiate sex, provide group identification for sexual subcultures, and resist the values of the hegemonic culture's categories were — and remain — largely untheorized.

Speaking of Sex . . .

While no government agencies were looking for opportunities to fund safe sex porn, *sexy* safe sex was promoted by extragovernmental agencies, like Jonathan Mann's policy think tank, the Harvard AIDS Institute, which advocated less didactic, more "explicit" campaigns using strategies extended from product marketing: *social* marketing might make condom use hip. But in the hands of agencies still aligned with the national pedagogy, sexually explicit images and ideas were decontextualized, produced as remedies to earlier failed safe sex interventions instead of connecting them organically to the evolving sexual subcultures. The national pedagogy refined its single narration of the compassionate citizen, but dissidents found it increasingly impossible to produce a unified narrative of safe sex that could encompass the wide range of identities and motives among men who had sex with men, much less among lesbians and other women with whom activists had hoped to ally themselves. The decade-long border war between the national pedagogy and dissident projects took on the quality of postcolonial crisis: even in the sexiest-looking campaigns, it was no longer easy to separate hegemonizing from dissident sexual advice.

Even the sexual definitions on which dissidents relied were no longer necessarily oppositional, or even solidly in the hands of those who asserted them.

Visualizing Safe Sex

As anxiety about object choice receded in the face of a discourse about aim, the national pedagogy was directed toward securing both heterosexuality's object and aim. A new "openness" about homosexual identity was now an essential ingredient in the national pedagogy: homosexuality might be a "natural" deviation of desire, but homosexual identity — or failing that, state identification of homosexuals — was required to ensure the stability of its object and aim, to prevent sodomites from "crossing over" into penetrative activities with women. Although they persisted, quasi-evangelical efforts to "reform" homosexuals to heterosexuality lost steam: not only could homosexuality be eliminated by leaving sodomites alone, but former homosexuals should be *prevented* from becoming "normal" if their conversion meant passing HIV to their "innocent" female partners. Although supposedly secular, the national pedagogy's explicit project to "promote behavior *change*" covered for a campaign to restabilize intercourse as a practice. The national pedagogy fueled the epidemic by engendering an ontological crisis: men — gay or straight — had to fuck more in order to demonstrate their choice of object.

The genocidal tendency that was only barely concealed in preepidemic psychiatry's abuse of homosexuals was replaced by an equally genocidal obfuscation. By constantly invoking intercourse as the aim to be deflected (as "safe sex") or channeled (as abstinence or monogamy), teaching the *nation* resulted in inciting queers — in two ways — to the very aim that was most hazardous: in order to sustain a "gay identity," or, in order to produce oneself as a sexual outlaw, gay men — especially young men — needed to refuse the "safe sex" that was held out as proper to the citizen: they had to "choose carelessly" (from the mainstream point of view) and refuse to fuck with a condom. The national pedagogy elaborated and magnified the necessity of intercourse and made it virtually impossible to articulate or represent sexual desire — aversive or attractive — in relation to anything else. To avoid intercourse was to drift into nondesire; to fuck with a condom was to accede to the undesirable, overdetermined program of the nation. The erotic subversiveness of having sex with *men* paled in comparison to the thrill of the antinationalist refusal to fuck with a condom. Thus, under cover of performing its duty, even while foisting "sexually explicit" campaigns on the public, the national pedagogy promoted the slaughter of two very different generations of gay men, along with male and female injecting drug users, and the women who had sex with either.[8]

Fatal Advice

138

Conclusion

From Visibility to Insurrection: A Manifesto

Throughout the 1980s, activists and educators experimented with increasingly provocative ways of promoting safe sex, but the national pedagogy met them at every turn. Influenced by intellectual trends that rigorously analyzed language — "texts" — safe sex activists overemphasized the power of a given text, while disregarding its uses in myriad places and its interpretation by multiple publics. The past year has brought renewed debate among activists about the failure of safe sex campaigns, along with renewed energy for finding better ways to reinvigorate transmission-interrupting sexual practices. Following the "in your face" visibility attained by ACT UP and Queer Nation, armed with renegade artists and activists with little interest in acquiring structural power, the new dissidence promises to challenge the national pedagogy in new ways. If they are to do more than thumb their noses at the national pedagogy, if they are to minimize the erosion of the spaces they hope to redefine, the new dissident educators and activists need to do more than produce shocking cartoons and confrontational slogans. They must develop better means of mobilizing the practical logics of erotic survival that already exist in communities, learn how and when these evolve in relation to the range of texts that intrude into or circulate beyond their borders. Reimagined sexualities — sexualities imagined beyond the nation — must become embedded in everyday life, not set apart as exceptional or extraordinary. Finding and using the implicit and explicit theories that inform the personal, political, and educational approaches to preserve the lives of sexual dissidents is not just an immediate project: *it is our lives.*

Charting a new course for saving our sexual culture will not be easy, precisely because our recent history is so tightly knit together with the articulation of late-twentieth-century American nationalism. It is not possible to step outside the political discourses and institutional compromises we have made. On the cusp of this new activism, we would do well to appreciate the reasons for past campaigns and neither vilify them for their failure nor discard them as proven unworkable. Condemning past activism will breed overoptimism about saving our sexual culture. Rejecting everything that has not yet worked means ignoring the context of past projects and potentially discarding strategies — including information campaigns — that might work differently now. It is important to see the next phase of organizing as a political project of queer survival, not as a mere correction for misguided ideas about safe sex. This requires linking the new organizing with its gay liberationist roots — but also recognizing that gay and lesbian organizing has diversified and evolved during the same time period, in relation to many, but not all, of the same forces. AIDS activism and gay activism are not the same thing, but saving sex requires a hybrid politics that can, finally, support each. We already know some of the problems that lie ahead: our notions of identity and community are at the heart of what must be radically rethought.

Uniting a new effort to save sex with the visibility and privacy tendencies in lesbian and gay politics is fraught with problems, the least of which is political incoherence. Talking out of both sides of our mouths, while it may seem to extend the issues we can take up and the coalitions in which we can participate, does not adequately address the need to preserve our erotic culture. But we need not adopt this dialectical framing of our political possibilities: we need not choose *between* visibility and privacy, *between* political space and the survival of desire, nor need we construct a shaky house with intersecting corridors composed from each. We must stop being obsessed with vision and space in these particular ways. The analogy to a cognitively oriented vision — one that requires us to see, understand, and name — no longer serves us. They have *seen* us already, and still, they do not understand what we mean with our self-naming. Likewise, the closet is an overworked, and increasingly impoverishing, spatial paradigm — we must either be in it, safe but claustrophobic, or out of it, proud, easier to target, agoraphobic. Instead, I want to argue for a notion that implodes vision into space, a space that may hold out more safety than either the closet or the light of day.

Broken down into its original Latin components, ob-scene adds a prefix indicating priority to scene, a root word meaning stage or theatrical place. Thus, ob-scene means something like *before staged* or indicates something before the moment of spatial visibility in official space. The implication is not so much a prior essence, or "real" to which a staging refers, but, simply, the before *here*. As a contemporary political idea, to put a spin on Baudrillard (1987), ob-scenity is the abjected, the meaningless, the thing that does not try to recover meaning but tries to secure the space *prior to visibility,* prior to information. Obscenity defeats the ideal of transparent communication that leaves us naked, but is required by the representational politics of the national pedagogy, and used, even still, by the dissident forces who have failed to defeat it. Ob-scenity is a kind of palpable presence that is not so much in-visible as it is detectable only on a different, potentially more disturbing, more *radical* level as a more deeply embodied volume. In some sense, the stead-fastly homophobic right (shockingly, even Newt Gingrich has said that most homosexuals on most days are upstanding citizens)[1] is already operating in this register of detection when they reject the idea that we can all live happily in our own little spheres, a minoritizing idealization of space that collapses the closet into privacy rights. They know that they will not rest safely until we are robbed of any space. We still don't want to admit that as long as we stay within liberal pluralism's idea of minority spaces, the reverse is also true. The only difference is that their capacity to eliminate us — directly through vio-lence and discrimination, or indirectly by interfering in the evolution of life-saving queer sex — is far greater than our capacity to circumscribe them.

Ob-scenity gives us another means of coming to terms with the current impasse between outing and privacy: we are only targets when we are visible, but that does not mean we have to be in a closet. Ob-scenity as politics, placing our bodies in an insurrectional posture prior to staging, *being here before,* offers a map composed through radically different coordinates. I want to gesture toward this new choreography of politics in the comments that conclude this book. Although I have been involved in numerous forms of queer dissidence since 1980, I have no answers, but I believe we have learned a few things. We must keep these in mind if we are to keep our friends and our desires alive through changing political and personal contexts, if we are to maintain the space of a truly subversive, perpetually critical and transforma-tive sex.

Conclusion

141

1. Sexuality emerges in action — participation in and observation of prohibitions and pleasures — and through "reading" — other bodies, medical texts, popular press accounts, how-to books, pornography. The particular matrix of participation, observation, and reading produces a range of positions in a variety of social spaces that create for each person a set of interpretive strategies that in turn position them in networks of policing, advice, possibilities, styles, erotic preferences, closets.

2. Sexual signification varies dramatically: elaborate systems are important in some cultures — many gay cultures, for example — and unimportant in others. Signification also varies by class, gender, ethnic group, age, location, and even time of day: flirting in the Star Market is not *doing* in the same way as cruising a bar later in the evening — even between the same interactants. Thus, determining appropriate use of sexual codes, or predicting how a set of sexual encodings will be interpreted, requires a complex understanding of registers of usage.

3. Thinking of sex as multiple vernaculars is a good antidote to a national pedagogy that presumes that language transparently communicates, rather than excludes, polices, incites. But linguistic and gestural signs don't primarily mean, they *do;* signs — words, moves, intuitions of desire — create space and guide action. Sex may well be the ideal perlocutionary system, more concerned with signing in order to get what you want than to have one's meaning understood as *meaning.* But the problem of making sex *save* is not that we fail to get across meaning — "fail to communicate" — but that the erotics of making-do are in themselves anticommunicative, are obscene in the strictest sense of that word. The power of safe sex discourse — the national pedagogy's *and ours,* until now — is that it demands obscenity as a response.

4. Sexual performance, what I prefer to call sexual vernacular, is contextual. The ways of being within sexual cultures are difficult to articulate, their processes of acculturation — their practices — are to some extent unspeakable, unformalizable.[2] Although sexuality is not only speech and gesture, desiring bodies are chiefly regulated through these: from psychiatry's attempt to elicit the hidden psychic language of deviant sexuality and then lobotomize, electroshock, or aversion therapize it from the brain, to queer

bashing that results from "reading" the victim as homosexual. Thus, defiant muteness about vernacular acculturation processes forms a critical line of defense for dissident sexualities. "Communicating" safe sex — as macroprojects called prevention campaigns or as the micro-inscription of individual erotic practice — does not transparently connect word with deed: a vernacular is intrinsically spatial, space and sexual signification are produced in and as power relations.

5. Understanding how a vernacular works requires identifying *how* values and concepts about sexuality and sexual practice have been effected within a community or micronetwork. The mediated and situated aspects of these symbolic processes — whether they are rap songs, dirty jokes, girl talk, how-to books — are the material templates for extending sex that saves our lives.

6. Space and identity converge in complex ways: a body names a place, a body takes names to a place, a body's presence transforms space — new names and a new sense of place arise. Vernacular is, therefore, a kind of tattered repository of the history of a place and the interplay of actors in it; an individual's ideolect — their peculiar combination of knowledges and signs — preserves the history of their trajectory through myriad spaces.

7. *Being* "in the life" precedes more visual markers of subcultural affinity. Those who are minimally bound together through a shared vernacular experience mutual recognition not so much through visual, ethnic-like marks, but when *what they say or how they move* makes body-sense to a potential sexual coenactant. Rich, elliptical sexual vernaculars characterize nomadic and unterritorialized sexualities.

8. The historical reality is that gay identity, as we know it, formed most visibly around white middle-class forms of same sex relations, and these are the ones that the media, politicians (including "our own"), and epidemiologists have also promoted as visible "gays and lesbians." People of color and men and women from other cultures and classes in which "bisexuality" is an unspoken norm are in jeopardy if mutual aid through "community" demands narrow identification with the white middle-class coming-out developmentalism that was critical for Western activism of the past two decades.

9. It may be strategically critical to continue asserting gay identity and gay community, but it is equally important to recognize that sexualities of resistance exist most importantly in their particularities of place and style, and

Conclusion
———
143

not in the adoption of particular identities and relations to communities that these identities imply. Sexual insurrection must work to open up sexual possibilities regardless of the names people choose for their pleasures.

10. All sexual spaces and forms have their rules of emergence and of practice, whether or not those who enter into them consider themselves to occupy a marked socio-sexual role. Sexual insurrection must sustain these unnamed sexual networks even while it reforms the consolidated, self-named gay community: ob-scene practices resist the increased social control over sexuality that jeopardizes the sex that protects us.

11. Only when a vernacular is raised to the level of official language in a political regime does it seem to be a natural or coherent language with a legitimate parentage. While heterosexualities have vernaculars, too, they are now primarily viewed as variations within the normative sexual category, minor deviations of aim. The governing metalanguage of heterosexuality uses its claim to naturalness — its simultaneous lack of vocabulary (who needs to talk about "it"?) and its totalizing logic (everything else is a fall from or perversion of bigender, penile-vaginal intercourse, and the presumption of an innate desire for "it") to intimidate those who operate in spaces marked by unhegemonized sexual vernaculars.

12. People from certain subgroups become afraid to speak their native tongue when their signs — a red hanky, a turn of phrase or cut of suit, a pamphlet, a book, an ideology — thought private suddenly come under scrutiny, become "public," rendering the internal language and symbols of a microculture vulnerable to unanticipated readings by an Other with greater discursive power. Members of the dominant language communities experience this publicizing theft (think of Jerry Falwell's direct mail pleas that foist pictures of queers on recipients) as an invasion of their ("private") territory by languages they do not wish to acquire. These dissident vernaculars may highlight, perhaps for the first time, the irregularity of border around dominant groups' arbitrary and unjustifiable coalitions of power.

13. The borders of microcultures are precarious, changing, co-opted by commercialism, and facilitated by the interpenetration of commercial cultures that camouflage minority desires. The live-and-let-live, peekaboo politic of pluralism will not protect us in a society penetrated by circulating capital. The money needed to produce pornographies rarely comes directly

from the communities who hope to use them. Mobile media threaten previous linguistic cordons (*Playboy* at the 7-Eleven; gay newspapers placed under surveillance and rendered as evidence in right-wing publications and in Congress). A curious ideology of taxation constructs the public will as a collectivity of purchasers — the appeal to "where your tax dollars go" made the Gay Men's Health Crisis pamphlet fair game for public debate over the content and style of a sexual language designed for "private" use within a community.

14. Hidden and legitimated languages of sexuality always collide, most often in contended social spaces. The idea of demarking public from private discourses as a means of protecting or limiting sexualities is not tenable. The supposed border between hegemonized and vernacular sexual significations is constantly eroding: dirty jokes, double entendres, and sexual leers slip out of bounds; medicalized discourses intrude upon the sexual (charts of Ronald Reagan's colon tumors may have done as much as the contemporaneous Surgeon General's report on AIDS to incite an aversive-obsessive attachment to anality); graffiti, euphemism, and pointed polite silence cross and explode the line between public and private. Countering the more powerful and obvious co-optation that occurs when vernacular fragments are incorporated into the national pedagogy, rapidly evolving slang both acknowledges and threatens the national silence.

15. Demarking acceptable and unacceptable language through literal zoning is a linguistic apartheid that quickly degenerates into administratively systematized genocide: dispersed in its landscapes of articulated sexualities, dominant society already contains the microcultures whose desires it would excise. Once partially protected as they reverberated beneath the range of audibility, surveys and medical examinations now wrest speech from — and linguistically quarantine — bodily pleasures that might easily save lives if they were not now condemned as dangerously perverse.

16. To say vernacular is "explicit" is only to recognize that for any group, phrases and gestures will have some conventional correspondence to concepts within the sexual imaginary and practices of the group. Thus, "sexual explicitness" is usually only registered as such by outsiders who tumble to the practical utility of terms or gestures that seem natural to those who routinely use them. Thus, explicitness has nothing to do with meaning, but with the

Conclusion
___

145

location of use and familiarity with a vernacular. Embarrassment or discomfort occur when the spatial limit of a group's vernacular is transgressed, when "the line" is crossed, but that line is specific to the group, and its relationship to other groups and to mainstream culture.

17. Sexually explicit material, deemed pornography by outsiders, is only vernacular formed within the interpretive scheme of a community or microgroup. There is not a spectrum with repressed sexuality on one end and liberated sexuality on the other, each with its own way of talking and moving. That pornography has been appealing as a mode of framing community concepts and values about "safe sex" among some sectors of the gay male community does not mean it will have utility for everyone, or even that every group should strive to create its own pornography. Rather, pornography is a vernacular for some networks of men and women: it "works," not because it is "explicit," accesses desire directly, or leaves no room for doubt, but because it is a richly ambiguous meditation on desire that makes sense among those who already recognize themselves in it.

18. If comprehended at all, most sexual vernaculars are offensive or embarrassing to those for whom it is not a native tongue. For different historical moments, Yiddish and Spanish ventriloquized the (English-obsessed) national culture's paranoid idea of the dangerously incomprehensible *foreign tongues* (as opposed to the useful, class-distinguishing French or Japanese). By contrast, sexual vernaculars, parasitic as they are on the dominant heteronormative language, are always already all *too* comprehendable. Reliant on found symbols and syntax, poaching, pastiching, or misaligning gestures from the heteronormative seduction repertoire, sexual vernaculars are especially open to misreading, provoking anxiety about the significance of *over*-familiarity more than xenophobia at foreignness.

19. Mere imitation or reproduction of a vernacular will not suffice; it may even be a dangerously subtle cultural imperialism. In order to be rich and useful to sexual cultures in transition, sexual cultures struggling with the requirements of the HIV epidemic — of the new homophobia, the new racism, the new sexism, the new "war on drugs" — a vernacular production must consider the *form* (oral, written, pictorial, gestural), *aesthetic,* and *mode of cultural circulation* of insurrectional ideas. The last is probably the least examined and the one most often violated in the quest for cultural sensitivity.

Fatal Advice

Outsiders can often catch on to the form and aesthetics of a vernacular, acquire a "second language" of sex, but rarely, or only after considerable trial and error, can they master the choreography, timing, and pathways of sexual performance that characterize a group or space.

20. Sex that saves lives is a cultural intervention that may work entirely within existing subcultural economies, or may stretch the edges of those economies, but cannot be imposed from outside. Activists must work within the conceptual logic of a group and must circulate within the borders of the microculture to renew and inform groups as they work through differing projects of renovated sexuality. There is an important difference between seeking the political/social visibility necessary to achieving rights and the spatio-symbolic safety we hope to extend as sexual vernaculars. The task of saving sex, of saving the bodies of desire, requires us to commit to each other, to risk exposing some of our way of life in order to form sexual cultures that resist both microbes and homophobes.

Spatializing Desire

I have spoken of this queer knowledge for more than a decade now, and I am often asked, "What should we do?" But while I have participated in many projects and offered advice on many others, we have to accept that no single formulation or plan will succeed in every place, every time. But armed with what we know, I want to offer a final suggestion for reimagining our sexualities as resistant, productive, *sexy*.

In the late 1980s, I grappled with how to improve safe sex campaigns and projects that I had helped design or that I had observed. Although I was highly critical of the idea of "communication," I was still overly concerned with language. I thought of the different kinds of projects as trying to effect change through different social formations of language — something like pidgin, Creole, and Esperanto seemed to capture the projects I knew. Pidgin seemed to represent the register of language used in places like cruising grounds, where men with divergent sexual identities (or none!) managed to get each other to perform pleasurable acts. Creole seemed to capture the emergence of identity, of coming from a place, of knowing fully a particular language that can only be used partially in a regularized space like a bar. Creole seemed to allow for

Conclusion
_____

147

multiple identities and desires, but attached them to the practicalities of finding sex and affection. Finally, Esperanto seemed to capture the transregionalization, even internationalization, of lesbian and gay identity, politics, and sexual styles: many of us can speak fluently in this artificial language, but it seems to have little to do with our desires.

While this scheme employed the key terms to which I believe insurgent forces must attend — relations of bodies, language, and space — they privileged language and a teleology of community development/identity formation that did not recognize the conflicts, separations, and retrograde motions of the sexualities I wanted to save.[3] Worse, the scheme did not easily capture the crucial dimension that a post–safe sex manifesto must include: desire. Language is sometimes part of an *ars erotica,* the thing that in part induces the acts to which it is presumed to refer. Instead, or also, we must think of body-language-space in productive terms, as erotic mobility: a vernacular is a hologram of the ways desiring bodies secure a place of sex/life.

Even at its most benevolent, the national pedagogy emphasized communication, the transparent verbalization of desire and technique, as a kind of contract. This in itself deeroticized the sex it hoped would be enacted under the sign of safe sex. It is not that talking ruins the mystery of the moment — for some it does, for others, talk is the sine qua non of their enacted desires — but that languaging safe sex under the avuncular national pedagogy was experienced as a kind of incestuous violation: safe sex is not boring to individual partners as much as it provokes a collective anesthesia at being fucked by the Uncle Sam who was supposed to protect us. Thus, I realized that my understanding of sexual space, of the languages we use, abuse, and misuse to define, protect, and direct others to the safe havens of our sex, required radical reorganization. I still feel there is merit in the general scheme, if only because the following elaboration seems to correspond to the spaces into which safe sex educators are trying to intervene. It is my hope that these parting comments will help us reconceive these spaces in ways that make us able to survive the rest of the 1990s.

Timing: A Sense of Where You Are

Public cruising areas are probably most obviously characterized as *place.* Viewed as communicative performances, cruising ground engagements are aimed at mutual recognition in a field of narrowly defined same sex action; they are pragmatic — aimed at accomplishing "sex." But to view them as lacking because they do not have a developed set of symbolic meanings that transcend the use of signs in particular spaces, that is, to only view them as pragmatic, indexical, not symbolic, or rich, discounts their porosity, their clever design that allows for quick provision of cover for "what a guy like me is doing in a place like this." Far from impeding the formation of a gay identity by sustaining male-male practice in an unchallenged netherworld of unreflexiveness, as some safe sex educators suggest, a cruising vernacular supplants the question of an abstract identification as "gay" with the certain "knowledge" of "where I am." The erotics of so-called "anonymous" sex relies on the pretence that participants do not know, or at any rate will not acknowledge, their relationships outside the hypopublic no man's land of cruising venues.

Thus, cruising vernacular is also act, structuring what sex *is, there.* The beautifully choreographed encounters in public cruising areas rely on gestures and clichés that may disgust outsiders, or offend insiders if used in another place (ostentatious crotch rubbing . . . at a cocktail party!). But framing cruising as only either communication or act overlooks the critical dimension of the cruising space — *timing,* the minute play of avowal and disavowal of intent, the choreography of desire that delimits and extends the "natural" boundaries of a cruising area. Time constitutes and defeats the perimeter of the park, the street names and traffic patterns, the entire toponymic grid imposed by the city's names, police districts, and rumors about areas. Cruising moves through the cruising ground but moves to and from homes and alleyways, creates smug recognitions and uncomfortable encounters when actants meet accidentally in some other place.

The minimalist vernaculars of cruising are used in specific types of encounters and marked by specific spaces (the park, bathhouse, etc.) or by a sign that converts a nondemarked space into a cruising area. The latter form of sign is especially dangerous — much more amazing than Wittgenstein's classic example of the customer trying to get the clerk to respond appropriately to the request for "red ones." Initiating and responding to cruising gestures puts the coordinative dimension of language to its test. In cruising, the body talks, it speaks its location, its intention, as it takes space. The situatedness of cruising, its bricoleur use of "found" fragments, means that the material markers

Conclusion
─────────

149

of its vernacular can also be discarded or defended as innocent. Artful cruisers can sometimes convince the police that they had no idea where they were. But a player who miscues, who takes another body to be desiring/it and inaugurates an elegant dance toward indexical conformity, risks the violence of heterosexuality's rebuke: death from queer bashing.

Queerbashers' readings rely on stereotypes from dominant culture — like effeminacy — or on a subculture's own evolving signs — being in a "gay" area or having a "gay" haircut — or simply on their conviction that they are desirable — their perception that a gay man has "cruised" them, even if what the victim did would not count as flirtation to a *gay* man. Thus, even cruising generates its vernacular in relation to a hostile dominant culture, even if its symbols are a kind of graffiti, a signature that defines a space by marking the absent presence of other homosexually desiring actors. To the extent that recognition and use of signs indicates membership, queerness is deeply tied to spatial claims. It is this slight oppositionality that begins to mark an individual who bears the knowledge of those codes, especially in responding to them. The fact of the cruising ground represents a potential: while everyone may know, on some level, *where* queers cruise, only a few people ever take advantage of their knowledge. But those who do not act cannot un-know and therefore can only disavow membership, they cannot *place* themselves elsewhere. In this sense, cruising areas are very much at the heart of heterosexuality's destabilization and not at all peripheral to it.

Queer Codes: Seeing Me/Seeing You

When people travel they carry — as a kind of body memory — the vernaculars that were vital to them in their myriad contexts. Although each vernacular evades attempts at codification, their elements "stick," even when the body that bears practical knowledge of them is not quite able to recognize a mark, gesture, or phrase as particular to a context through which it has passed. A swagger, a certain cut of hair, a look, a phrase: these sticky elements, when detached from their place of maximum practical utility, become queer codes. Where cruising vernaculars served as ritual shorthands that to some extent foreclosed reflexive communication about the sexual encounter, and did not invite philosophical comment on the meaning of the encounter, travel begins to introduce and enact notions of space memory, of membership. Making a miscue while cruising resulted, on one hand, in failure to get what one desired — sex or companionship of some kind — or, in the tragic scenario, in violent retaliation by a homophobe. Languages that have traveled raise issues of legitimacy: mistakes in queer codes cause suspicion among those who feel proprietary interest in a vernacular.

Cruising out of context is read as crudeness; by association, displaying a queer code announces the user as a member of a subculture, at least to other members of that group. Cruising vernaculars exist in and for — and even define — particular places: queer codes define a network of participants and enable them to mobilize a collective memory — of past sexual episodes and queer spaces — when elsewhere. Queer codes define *as* a *space* the linkage between interlocutors who recognize that they know and share a particular sexual vernacular, can use it even under the eyes of people who might harm them if they recognized the associative significance of the vernacular ("signifyin' "). Use of queer codes is common among gay/lesbian-identified people who can quickly "check out" the membership of others without nonmembers even recognizing that an erotic linkage has occurred in the middle of a conversation in which they participated. While the structure and common strategies of contemporary gay/lesbian codes are often recognized by sensitive nonmembers, imitation reveals interlopers as nonnatives to them. But poor fidelity may be purposeful: it is interesting to me that straight people are less inclined to display their knowledge of queer codes than white people are inclined to display their knowledge of black codes. Could it be that use of queer codes always risks transforming the present space into a cruising ground, while use of black codes by whites only redraws the line between the races?

Queer codes require some recognition of symbolic relationships related to sexuality that are beyond the pragmatics of a sexual negotiation: they introduce the possibility of establishing unconscious associations between language and the "truth" of an interior sexuality, of misrecognizing the stickiness of accumulated vernacular as essence.[4] Thus, the belief that individuals' articulations of queer codes are evidence of a particular psychic sexual structure misrecognizes the code user's status as a participant in a subgroup that has generated the code as a means of securing protective systems of mutual

Conclusion
-----

recognition. What we think of as the "unconscious," the reservoir of desire that can be repressed, incited, or revolutionized, is really the name for spaces of bodily enactment that are carried as marks and memories.

Hyperspace: Cruising the Imagined Community

Queer codes gain cultural weight as they are increasingly produced and understood as representations of gay/lesbian individuals. The "secret" that pathologized homosexuality, that placed a traumatic burden on the individual who possessed it, is now the responsibility of those in the dominant culture who refuse queer presence. The prosaic similarity in "coming out" stories, ritually recounted within sexual communities, represents not a psychic similarity in homosexual desire/identity, but the political accomplishment of a translocal narrative form. The coming out story universalizes and individuates lesbians and gay men as bodies produced through the collision of social repression and the natural forces of desire. This "explanation" of lesbian and gay existence is now part of the national cultural, however precariously: the coming out story is the quintessential "true self" hermeneutic, a melodramatic account of essence and self-discovery.

The emergence of a lively and diverse gay and lesbian press and the acceptance within some liberal periodicals (largely as a result of AIDS) of stories from the point of view of lesbians and gay men have created additional structures for encoding and communicating sex. Available for use by bodies with no other relation to spaces of queer production, a third kind of subcultural language had emerged by the mid-1980s, a kind of Esperanto linking imagined national and international communities of bodies who interpret themselves as sharing something in common (though *what* is not exactly clear). Gay people are extremely good at decoding messages about or aimed at us in everything from descriptions about "risk reduction" ("avoiding exchange of fluids" is clearly directed toward gay men, whose penetrative reversibility might be described as "exchange" in a way that heterosexual intercourse can only count as a "deposit") to obituaries (a young age combined with respiratory failure, cancer, or a "long illness," sealed by the lack of a surviving wife). While these trace the perimeter of a queer world, of imagined communities that only partially subsume the desires and recognitions of cruising and queer codes, they are remarkable in their avoidance of pragmatic, "sexual" address.

Thus, while not entirely visible, this transnational vernacular of gay liberation is not exactly ob-scene. Indeed, this is the trait of our Esperanto: its degree of visibility makes us uncomfortable using it for the conduct of desire, makes it capable of speaking *for* all of us — as a *movement* — without speaking *to* any of us. Yet, this is the register in which much "safe sex" is propagated — and probably conducted. (No wonder once exciting activities have become boring under the new safe sex Esperanto!) Commercial pornography has to some extent filled (and exploited) the gap left by the gay and lesbian movement's avoidance of speaking in locally erotic *sexual* vernaculars. The requirements of global organizing despatialized homodesires in the very act of transnationalizing an apparently universal gay and lesbian identity and speech. Despite its hopes of staging mass presence through a political-public language with global appeal, this only regularized the kinds of speech that the right wing called pornographic. Even academically legitimated discussion of sexuality could not be secured: in 1993, the weighty tome of essays collected as the *Lesbian and Gay Studies Reader* (Abelove, Halperin, and Barale 1993) was seized as obscene under the Canadian law modeled after the failed American MacKinnon ordinances.

All sexual vernaculars are complexly linked to the dominant language system and its ability to police the borders of spaces that sexual vernaculars, in their various ways, inscribe. Nonetheless, there are important differences in the forms of queer inscription that reflect the motivations and identification of the speakers. Our battle to make our sex safe requires protecting *all* of these forms, which will require activisms of very different sorts. Civil rights activism can save jobs and homes and save lives by extending social programs and making visible the violence and discrimination against sexual dissidents. But political projects are no more an essential source of our presence than are our desires: we should take them up or put them down, activate or redirect them like tools or machines. Whatever skepticism I have about the possibilities, in the current climate, for civil rights successes, I am unwilling to abandon such legible efforts, though they are in urgent need of new rhetorics. But I am no more certain that current anarchist or oppositional forms actually confront, rather than merely reconstruct, their enemies.

Conclusion

I will reveal my political bias: the recent New Right takeover of Congress under the gentle night of Republicanism only presses on us the urgency of being *more* not *less* evidently antinational. However important they were in their moments, "SILENCE=DEATH" and "queer nation" now mean only that a chatty nation loves its fashionable queers — to death. "Activism" must go beyond the New Left-style call to "Organize!" and must instead launch a full-scale insurrection. This assault must unite "academics" and "activists" — not as a peace-making mission, but because a fully ob-scene, rather than civilly visible or reactively closeted, political strategy requires a combination of the brazen perversions of queer theory and the brutally achieved queer street knowledge. We will never find — should not even seek — a unified political language, but we can learn to operate in a range of mutually untranslatable, intrinsically differently motivated vernaculars. Sometimes we must make sense to government agents, but we shouldn't confuse this reeling moment of apparently transparent communication with a true recognition of queer presence by forces who generally oppose us.

Insurrections capable of making sex safe (from disease *and* social repression) do not require recruiting everyone to gay identity. Demanding a narrow and historically constructed understanding of identity not only misunderstands the political importance of diversities in sexuality, but relinquishes the particular strengths that obtain among same sex practitioners who go under other names. This does not at all mean giving up the communities that have achieved strength and visibility as positively lesbian and/or gay, but to accept the idea that everyone else is duplicitously "in the closet" is to hand over tremendous political power to the state. Heterosexism demands that we name partners and limit sexuality to a narrow range of cross-gender behaviors. To demand a narrow gay identity — even implicitly, as in safe sex educational campaigns — runs the risk of duplicating this form of oppression. To refuse to claim that everyone any of us has ever had sex with is thereby "gay" is not to degay our community: rather, it is to complicate and confound heterosexuality, to create more space for sexual alliances, not less. Reclaiming sexual spaces and subcommunities on their own terms builds on the strength of queer culture without ceding the specific history and gains of urban gay communities — they are a vitally important form of queer culture, and one uniquely positioned to channel resources from the state to projects that save our lives. But they are not the only form.

Fatal Advice

Perhaps ironically, I close this genealogy of safe sex with a final spin on Baudrillard's concept of fatality: readers will forgive me for concealing the motivating pun until this last breath. Yes, the advice given by the national pedagogy has killed more people than it has saved; we number among the fatalities those we have known and loved, those whose faces we have never seen, whose names we'll never hear, and yes, we even number *ourselves*. But we can turn the tables, not through a direct opposition, but through pulling the plug on advice, through living our desires as a sex that saves instead of finding and vilifying people and practices that do not.

The next step may be to stop using the term "safe — even safer — sex" and to reject any idea of a wholesome "gay lifestyle." Instead, we must think about sex as the form of power that makes and saves queer lives. This requires us to stop defining and promoting an object, *a* sex that can be categorically distinguished from its multiple Others, the ones that are sustained as dangerous, deadly, etc. There is only *one* dangerous act, being fucked without a condom, that sole act, not coincidentally, which is invoked by the national pedagogy as the citizen's "freedom" — having license to *fuck without a condom* is the new, all-American fantasy of heterosexuality rescued from queerness.

But we must do more than mobilize dissident bodies against the doubly and truly fatal homo-annihilation project of the national pedagogy. We must figure out how to recruit the multiplicity of queer desires to life in a new dimension of political effectivity. The twin, if paradoxical, projects of visibility and privacy have nearly run their course: neither can save us. Our next sexual politic *must* be ob-scene.

Conclusion

Notes

1. Around 1989

1. The occasion of this paper was the first lesbian and gay studies conference held at Yale University. The paper was published as "Hegemony and Orgasm, or the Impossibility of Heterosexuality," *Screen,* 1990.

2. The "come shot" or "money shot" is the spectacular display of male orgasm.

3. Safe sex pamphlets do not recommend this technique since most men cannot reliably "pull out" before ejaculation, and because some men have copious quantities of pre-come, also potentially implicated in HIV transmission.

4. The regionally distributed newspaper *GO* was published by the Gays of Ottawa, the local gay and lesbian council, but was governed by a partially autonomous editorial board. *GO* was somewhere between a house publication and an independent newspaper, two media that had figured prominently in the formation and interconnection of geographically dispersed gay and lesbian communities of the twentieth century. Both forms had been especially crucial during the first years of the epidemic, when mainstream media declined to say anything about HIV prevention or care. The ad in question had been approved by the lesbians and gay men of the editorial board, folks savvy about local political trends.

5. Indeed, I've long argued that opposing gay men's and women's interests hampers the feminist agenda more than it helps it. Although it is not always easy to form happy coalitions across deeply gendered issues, policy and research logics, and not individuals' prejudices, frame the categories of visibility and urgency that are responsible for small groups' need to fight over meager resources. See especially my *Last Served? Gendering the HIV Pandemic* in which I argue that gendered ideologies overdetermine

the categories into which "men" and "women" are placed for policy, research, and educational purposes.

6. Louis Althusser's (1977) famous formulation of "interpellation" argues that people come to their identity and sense of place in the world because the various ideologic dimensions of a monolithic state "hail" them as the sort of person the state wants them to be. This is figured as the citizen who, while walking down the street, is hailed by the policeperson: the citizen turns because, despite not hearing her or his name, he or she simply *knows* that the policeperson is addressing them.

7. I develop this idea of identity more extensively in the forthcoming "Refiguring Social Space" (1995).

8. Eve Kosofsky Sedgwick (1990) popularized the terms *universalizing* and *minoritizing* within gay and lesbian studies. These refer to the basic logics of post-Stonewall gay thought, roughly, that people are polymorphously perverse or queer in different ways and by degrees, or by contrast, that only a set proportion of the population desire members of the same sex and these constitute a minority. The first leads to politics that diminish sharp lines between forms of sexuality. The latter leads to civil rights, which stabilize the mark of difference in order to demonstrate and historicize harm and clearly distinguish those who should be protected or given a remedy. Lisa Duggan's 1992 "Making It Perfectly Queer" is an excellent mapping of the essentialism/social construction debates that brought 1980s activism to its identity crisis — or crisis over identity. Henry Abeloves's (1994) "From Thoreau to Queer Politics" suggests that queerness and its identification as such were fundamental to American politics such as those expressed in Thoreau's *Walden.* My preface to the republication of *Lavender Culture* also provides a general overview of the problematics of 1970s gay thought and the disingenuousness of some contemporary interpretations of it.

9. One of the most damaging features of debates about the relative safety of various possible sexual activities is the suggestion that, somehow, there are new or yet to be discovered "facts" that will substantially affect what we know about how to avoid becoming infected. The only major changes concern fellatio — still hotly debated, but most likely much safer than early advice suggested — and female-to-male transmission, which, though we early knew that it is a difficult and relatively minor route, continues to be asserted as a significant source of danger to men during heterosexual intercourse.

10. These included relatively unreported acts of violence against gay men and prostitutes, as well as highly publicized accounts of the burning of the Ray family home in Florida and the exclusion of Ryan White from his elementary school.

11. The Justice Department declared that discriminating against a person thought to have AIDS was excusable if done out of ignorance, but not if the discriminator knew the "facts," an executive branch order that complicated a Supreme Court decision, handed down only months earlier, that discrimination based on fear of perceived disease violated statutes concerned with disabilities.

Notes

12. Earlier versions of some of the work here appeared as "Visualizing Safe Sex: When Pedagogy and Pornography Collide," in *Inside/Out: Essays in Lesbian and Gay Theory,* ed. Diana Fuss (New York: Routledge, 1991); "Safe Sex and the Pornographic Vernacular," in *How Do I Look?,* ed. Douglas Crimp (Seattle: Bay Press, 1991); "Designing Safer Sex: Pornography as Vernacular," in *A Leap in the Dark: AIDS, Art and Contemporary Cultures,* ed. Allan Klusacek and Ken Morrison (Montreal: Vehicule Press, 1992); and "Fear of AIDS: Innocence and Ingenuity," *American Imago,* Fall, 1992; and "Between Innocence and Safety: Representations of Young People's Need to Know about 'Safe Sex,'" *Deviant Bodies,* ed. Jacqueline Urla and Jennifer Terry (Bloomington: Indiana University Press, 1995).

13. Because of men's greater economic power and their strong position in the arts, homoerotic male nude photography began with the first experiments in photography. The pretense of physique magazines, popular among gay men in the mid–twentieth century, enabled some gay men to cultivate erotically pleasing images without completely running foul of the law. Lesbians had parallel, but much less developed, spaces for producing or appropriating erotic media — especially the cheap lesbian pulp novels of the same era. Although the covers of these novels had a well-established visual code, lesbians seemed to have developed a more articulate verbal code. This picture-word split seems to continue in current commercial and noncommercial lesbian and gay erotic works.

14. I am only sketchily describing a complex and bitter political battle about sexuality. For more extensive discussion see Duggan and Hunter (1995), who bring together analysis of specific campaigns regarding sexuality — especially the pornography debates — under the concept of sexual dissent. They reformulate the debates about sexuality as essentially political battles for the capacity to disagree with what is, though often covertly, national or governmental policy regulating sexuality. This framework, along with Jonathan Dollimore's (1991) conception of nonhegemonic sexualities as intrinsically and politically dissident, has significantly influenced my own evolution from seeing radical safe sex work as oppositional to seeing it as part of a larger structure of ongoing dissidence.

15. The national pedagogy relies on the hypodermic model of information exchange. The ease with which people claimed that information is a vaccine evokes Baudrillard's contention that increasing information evacuates meaning.

16. On her controversial sitcom, Roseanne kisses a lesbian character — Mariel Hemingway — who appears as the occasional girlfriend of series regular Sandra Bernhard. When challenged by Bernhard, Roseanne responds that she isn't *gay,* is maybe a few percent gay, but, she reasons, everyone is a little bit gay. In this common logic of polymorphous perversity, one must be gay in larger quantities in order to be truly gay.

17. For example, the late 1980s saw another form of national pedagogy that sought

Notes

159

to reconstruct the body of the citizen: the massive and aggressive "low fat" campaign. The AIDS campaigns and the antifat campaigns were, in fact, interestingly at odds, even though in both cases, "risk" was held out as a call to responsibility. But while the antifat campaigns, finally waged in collaboration with the food industries, used a population-wide strategy, the adoption of universal precautions was never viewed as a threat to the nation, as was the possibility of universal condom use in the case of HIV prevention.

The attempts to decrease coronary heart disease are also an interesting example of how campaigns can, over time, shift from risk-based to population-based strategies, especially if new consumer markets can be created. Until the past two decades, decreasing risk of coronary heart disease was largely left up to the individual who had already begun to show symptoms. Research in the 1970s resulted in delineation of risk formulas (overweight, family history, smoking, etc.), which individuals could use to determine whether they should modify their lifestyle by exercising or eating "dietetic" foods, which were banished to a special and limited shelf in the supermarket. The 1980s saw a shift in social mores and in food research; moderate exercise was advocated for everyone and new, better-tasting low-fat foods not only appeared, but in some cases almost completely replaced older products now perceived to have unnecessary amounts of cholesterol. The shift from efforts to identify and dietetically punish those at particular risk to decreasing cholesterol consumption and increasing the exercise level of everyone was complete, but it required a major shift in the popular concepts and media representation of exercise (for example, walking now counts) and "healthy food," including integration of such products onto the regular shelves in the supermarket. Clearly, the social costs and economic benefits of particular styles of health education extend far beyond the physician's office. Whole industries rise and fall based on research interests in and marketing of "health" and health beliefs. Attempts at condom marketing might have helped shift HIV prevention education to a population-wide strategy; however, social mores (television wouldn't air ads, it was difficult to get the product sold at likely outlets — schools, vending machines, publicly funded clinics) thwarted even capitalism's attempts to enter a new health promotion market.

18. The "AIDS doesn't discriminate" campaigns were catchy, but the idea of preventing transmission imploded in the face of a logic that suggested that compassion was something like a virus: if "it" doesn't discriminate, neither should I. Alternatively, the common belief that heterosexuals should "choose carefully" suggested that "it" doesn't, but you should. The national pedagogy found a delicate balance between these paradoxes: people should discriminate on the individual, sexual level, but not on the social level. Clearly, this presumed a sharp separation between domestic and civic affairs.

19. I believe that distinguishing between HIV and AIDS is crucial not only to laying the foundation for understanding the scientific information about the syndrome, but

Notes
———
160

also for building good reasoning for making decisions about transmission interruption and about medical care, if one is infected. However, the media undercut its own attempts to make the distinction by suggesting that it is a semantic detail of little consequence to the reader, a kind of technical correctness that has little real impact. Once they had trained Americans to correctly use the terms HIV and AIDS, they should have made it clearer why the virus versus syndrome distinction matters. I believe that most lay people still think through policy decisions as if HIV and AIDS were the same.

20. This rider to the enabling legislation, which allows AIDS funding categories to be automatically renewed each year with new amounts of money, denied funding to campaigns that "promote" homosexuality and promiscuity.

21. Indeed, many people called this the second epidemic, again displacing gay liberationist and feminist critiques of heterosexism by situating the cause of ill treatment of people living with AIDS in individual ignorance about "difference," rather than pursuing larger and more systemic arguments.

22. The current debates about risk reduction need to recognize this element in the history of safe sex. Dissident educators who wish to continue this tradition must recognize that the national pedagogy has been successful in insisting that one is required to tell one's serostatus. Even in the gay community, men have many reasons for telling and not telling: it is not possible to assume that they are not asking or telling because the universal safe sex strategy has prevailed. Men both fail to practice safe sex out of assuming a partner who doesn't say anything is *not* placing them at risk and do practice safe sex (by simply never practicing intercourse) without realizing they have done so without needing to know another's serostatus. The problem of not disclosing one's serostatus comes about because a specific meaning is attached to saying nothing, and a decision-making process is set into motion based on that meaning. The idea that you can tell if someone is seropositive by looking (still, I believe, a prevalent belief — many gay men simply believe they have a larger pool on which to base such "educated" guesses) is partially replaced by the idea that you can tell their status by whether they disclose it or by what they will agree to do. In this logic, those who don't tell you they are seronegative are suspicious (but really, wouldn't that be the more dangerous lie to believe?) while those who refuse to disclose and instead practice safe sex are assumed to be positive (but really, aren't they avoiding the possibility of everyone's lies?)

The other crucial difference in sex between men concerns its reversibility and the complex moral identifications that this seems to have created. In truth, the receptive partner — like his female physiologic counterpart — is at far greater risk of infection . . . and of cultural scorn for being queer. Several sensational accounts of practicing unsafe sex, which appeared in New York newspapers in the spring of 1995, confuse the biomechanics of risk with the outrage of being — and placing others — at risk of HIV transmission. These accounts seem to be by seronegative men who were the insertive

Notes

161

partners with men who did not disclose their serostatus. On one hand, the risk to themselves, if the receptive partner was positive, is very low. If the confessors to unsafe sex had in fact been seropositive, *their* actions would have placed their partners at high risk of becoming infected, if they were seronegative (reinfected, or coinfected it they were already seropositive).

For better or worse, knowledge (real or imaged) of serostatus has become a significant part of gay men's process of deciding when and how to have sex. Although I still believe that a universal safe sex model is, in the long run, better than various kinds of partner selection models (including those based on serostatus), activists who want to continue this strategy must now accept and work with the apparently haphazard ask-and-tell structure that seems to be normative at least in some cities like New York.

23. It was because gay men's groups so badly needed funding that the most public clash over how to do safe sex education occurred. In 1987, Sen. Jesse Helms of North Carolina displayed on the floor of the Senate some sexually explicit, culturally sensitive brochures from the Gay Men's Health Crisis in New York City. The particular pamphlet that drew the most ire was a cartoon book about S/M sexuality by a gay artist whose style was immediately recognizable to gay men from this "hard to reach" urban subculture. Helms argued that American tax dollars had paid for the booklet. It didn't matter that Helms was wrong — the scrupulous bookkeeping of groups like GMHC easily showed that these kinds of projects had been supported from private funds. Nevertheless, Helms was able to leverage personal distaste into political terrorism. Numerous AIDS service agencies were harassed by right-wing legislators who demanded audits of financial records and of materials produced by the group.

24. During my two years as an ethnographer at several methadone clinics, I discovered that there are all sorts of misunderstandings about receiving test results. Many people test but do not return for results, believing that if they are seropositive, the clinic will call them. Others donate blood, again presuming that if they are found to be seropositive the donation center will contact them. Finally, many people engage in a complex calculus I think of as surrogate testing, in which one member of a sexual network tests and, if they test negative, the others assume they must be negative, too.

25. Of course, it took several years of study — approximately until 1988 or 1989 — before epidemiologists could narrow down the "window period," i.e., the length of time from infection to actually mounting a detectable antibody response. The idea that a negative test, especially two or more, constituted a "clean" bill of health was solidly in place before scientists achieved consensus on average seroconversion times.

26. Certainly, knowledge of antibody status affects individuals in a wide variety of ways, related to health beliefs, social and psychological support, community attitudes, to suggest only a few. Before there was clear evidence for use of *pneumocystis carinii* pneumonia (PCP) prophylaxis in particular, and, controversially, zidovudine (AZT), many gay community groups opposed widespread testing, especially if the principal

Notes

purpose was to change behavior. By the end of the 1980s, there were renewed calls for testing, this time with the support of the gay community, now with hopes that asymptomatic people could take advantage of treatments. But, with the exception of PCP prophylaxis and some treatments for specific coinfections, there were no clear medical advantages to learning that one was seropositive before becoming symptomatic: the calls for early testing collaborated uneasily with the compassionate release of zidovudine and its less toxic analogues. The invocation to "do no harm" lost out to fears of withholding potentially effective (though unproven) treatments. There may also have been a collision between doctors' increasing fear of malpractice and activists' desires to assume the risk of unapproved treatments. In essence, calls for early antiviral intervention for asymptomatic people (as opposed to symptomatic people, many of whose symptoms could be treated with existing or modified drugs) came well before there was clear evidence that early medical intervention was successful at altering the course of HIV disease. Indeed, the European Concorde studies initiated and producing results during the same time period as the U.S. trials suggested that zidovudine-type antivirals provided no advantage in long-term survival rates for those treated early. Although individuals may have benefited from enrolling in trials, I think it is fair to say that mass testing — first wrongly presumed to be a motivator of behavior change — became an only marginally ethical mechanism for enrolling research subjects. By creating the hope that early intervention could prolong life, antibody testing protocols created a demand for the still equivocal antiviral drugs. The promotion of "education as the only 'vaccine'" doubled the logic of promoting clinical trials as "the only hope."

2. Between Innocence and Safety

1. Estimating the number of people living with HIV is extremely complex; the usually cited ratio of ten seropositives to each diagnosed case of AIDS is an equivocal figure, dependent on the amount of "surveillance" (testing) of a community and the representativeness of those tested, on evolving effectiveness of treatments to slow the progression of symptoms that qualify as AIDS, on the varying longitudinal success of behavior change, on the timing of measurement in relation to the epidemic curve (the longer a community has been at or near "saturation," the lower the ratio of infected to diagnosed people), and on little understood factors like biological variations in susceptibility to infection if exposed.

2. Burroughs-Wellcome is the manufacturer of zidovudine (AZT) and one of the largest providers of information to non-gay-oriented clinics providing HIV antibody counseling and testing.

3. This line of argument was common in far-right publications. Some went so far as

Notes

163

to claim that safe sex was a plot to produce heterophobia and distrust between the sexes. See Antonio (1986).

4. The quarterly *Youth and Society* emerged as and continues to be a major locus for academic work from this theoretical frame. Instead of the individualistic approach of psychology and social psychology that, while challenging the storm and stress model on empirical grounds, nevertheless takes the plight of the individual young person as the object of study, the subcultural approach uses the methods of anthropology and qualitative sociology to study either clusters of youth or the concept of youth itself. For example, a typical study of sexual attitudes and behavior among youth (Miller, Christensen, and Olson 1987) rejects social-psychological concepts like "self-esteem" and parental "permissiveness" as useful ways to understand teen pregnancy. Instead, the authors argue that both parental and teen attitudes depend on cultural context, in particular, on the subculturally specific symbolic meaning of virgin versus nonvirgin status and on codes about sex itself.

5. After a year of rumors that he was gay, or that his dance career had been stalled because he had AIDS, Ron Reagan, Jr., was also featured in one of the group's films discussing safe sex for heterosexuals.

6. The issue of racial constructions of audiences is extremely complex in U.S. entertainment and news media because of the long history of slavery in which whites both feared black insurrection and made blacks perform entertainments that featured insurrection and punishment. Real whippings were an entertainment staple on plantations, and theatrical whippings continued to be popular with white audiences of minstrel theater. The combination of paranoia and desire to possess other cultures produced a complex sequel: whites like to pretend to peer over the shoulder of entertainment blacks produce for themselves. With the increase in mass media, it is now often impossible to tell the racial demographics of the actual audience of apparently black or black-aimed productions. Whites may not understand black-aimed productions in the same way as their "target" audience, but they have long-standing means of insinuating themselves as a voyeuristic audience, and take great pleasure in having "inside" knowledge of a culture whose producers they otherwise dislike, discriminate against, and fear.

3. The Erotics of Innocence

1. I want to be clear that I do not review the Freudian account because I believe it is *the* truth of sexuality, but because it seems to be the major narrative underlying the contemporary discourse of innocence.

2. In recent years, kiddie porn cases have worked in tandem with the highly pub-

licized day-care molestation cases: men whose pornography collections are used as evidence against them are assumed to have done in mediated form what day-care center operators are alleged to have done in person. While child empowerment is a worthy project, the protectionist rhetoric and overactive policing in the high-media-profile cases are antifeminist and homophobic. The day-care hysteria seems less de-signed to enable children to protect themselves than it is aimed at policing working mothers by representing them as heartless women who jeopardize their children by putting them in institutional care in order to pursue their own careers. The kiddie porn cases represent their young victims as the fallout of the sexual revolution, either runaways from broken families or kidnappees of sexual libertarians. While there are certainly ruthless individuals in both cases, it would seem that the fault lies not with feminists or sexual liberationists, but with capitalist social arrangements, which fail to provide adequate care for children of workers and neglect the interests of young workers themselves.

3. Public health officials, "victims," and civil litigants have had extreme difficulty establishing a *legal* obligation to know or reveal one's HIV antibody status, not least because the modes of transmission are largely voluntary practices and the means of prevention so technically easy for either party. Given the difficulty individuals outside the hardest hit groups (urban gay men and urban drug injectors) have recognizing their own risk, and given that test taking does not reliably stimulate risk reduction, it seems particularly hazardous to hang the safety of heterosexual sex on the very innocent expectation that one's partner will be willing and able to accurately share test results. Here, the sexual innocence attributed to adolescence has percolated upward and has destructively misshaped the "adult messages" regarding safe sex practices.

4. "The Only Weapon We Have . . ."

1. See Patton (1990). Because a basic moral ambivalence about the activities that enable transmission remains, researchers have argued in favor of using placebo-controlled vaccine trials on groups held to be intransigent to advice because they are illiterate or impoverished, or because their sex drive is considered "unstoppable."

2. These included "lifestyle" features that we now know may affect progression of HIV illness, but have nothing to do with initial infection. This basic confusion remains in social science research on risk and in advice on how to avoid it. Terms like "risk situation" and "risk relevant behavior," while useful in fleshing out the social context in which transmission might occur, continue to be confused with the biological proper-ties of the virus and the fluids in which it travels.

3. David Roman pointed out to me that several of the early AIDS benefits, hosted by

Notes

165

communities large and small during the early 1980s, raised money to be sent to emerging AIDS groups in the major cities to which the smaller cities felt related.

4. The proliferation of Knowledge, Attitude, (Behavior,) and Practices (KAP or KABP) studies worldwide produced the perception that we understand sexuality and sexual behavior. This form of scientific research has become an institution in itself, pulling research on sexuality and on descriptions of local risk toward quantitative study that will inevitably produce information and behavior change campaigns that are oriented toward individuals. They also engender individualistic evaluation of the pre-test/posttest form, which tells nothing about the process through which any change has occurred, much less how to achieve normative changes over the long haul. Despite continual criticism of the paucity of this kind of study, once it is established as the mark of local knowledge and the first step in the development of campaigns, it is difficult to convince funding agencies to support other forms of research.

5. Whatever the numerical realities of gay men and lesbians' sexual compulsion and drug addiction, the rise in concern about excesses of pleasure marched lockstep with the mainstream, Reaganite views on drugs and sex. Some AIDS educators made an effort to articulate drug and alcohol abuse as an effect of homophobic oppression rather than a symptom of individual pathology, but this view was difficult to apply to sex without appearing to claim that gay men were in some essential way self-destructive, a position that groups designed to deprogram homosexuals had already taken. After identification of the virus, overload hypotheses that had linked AIDS with designer drugs and poppers (amyl nitrate) faded. Partly because they were misled by epi-demiologists' failure to describe more clearly the dual-route category of gay injecting drug users (around 20 percent), by the mid-1980s the gay community generally viewed *sex* as the most important link with HIV/AIDS: sex was both the precondition for the epidemic and the mechanism — as *safe* sex — for stopping it. Like their straight peers in chemical dependency counseling (of the non–twelve-step variety), most saw sex as controllable and promoted safe sex rather than abstinence. A minority, however, viewed sexual compulsion as the problem underlying the viral epidemic — without compulsive sexual behavior, they reasoned, the epidemic would not have become so extensive. For those whose analysis was centered on sexual compulsion, things that promoted and celebrated sex — in particular, pornography and the traditional cruising venues — were dangerous for the sex addict. But in general, the hardline addiction view was more often applied to drug use than to sex, and sexual compulsiveness was less accepted as an issue than substance abuse: lesbian and gay substance abuse was treated as a separate, *non*-HIV health issue. Indeed, the ad for a major gay-operated detox and therapy center (Pride Institute) argued that more gay people die each year from "chemical dependency" than from AIDS, a claim that rested on a logic that angered many AIDS activists — that the "new" problem of AIDS had displaced more

Notes
———

important, long-standing gay issues. This also obscured what turns out to be the most significant risk for lesbians. Reanalysis of data from several major drug studies suggests that there are small networks of women who have sex primarily with women who also share needles primarily with women. Targeted neither through their sexual identity, nor through their drug use (the vast majority of injectors are men and education has been directed to them and their female partners), these women have much higher rates of infection than their female peers who have sex with and share needles with men. Thus, lesbian injectors are at higher risk because their microcommunities have gone untargeted by educators because lesbians in general were not perceived to be at risk. That is, they are at higher risk because they live outside the intensively educated gay male and injector communities, due to their sexual identifications but not because of their sexual practices.

5. Visualizing Safe Sex

1. John d'Emilio (1984) details the pre-Stonewall legal cases in which physique magazines favored by gay men and the early gay periodicals were seized by the U.S. Postal Service. Since Stonewall, gay materials have been consistently the object of local and international censorship as obscene.

2. These included me, then Manager of Community Education and acting Co-director of the Education Department of the AIDS Action Committee of Massachusetts; Steven Colarusso, also an Education Department staff member; and longtime volunteers Chris LaCharite and Sandy McLeod. There was no one in the gay male educator job at the time, and the AAC was in the process of downsizing. There was extreme disagreement about how to conduct gay male education, and the number of education volunteers had dropped to almost zero by the time I was hired. As a volunteer-initiated project (Chris and Sandy had been working toward such a project for some months before my arrival), which was then solidly backed by a senior staff member who had fairly wide credibility in the local community, the project provided a bridge between agency-owned and truly community-based programming. In line with AAC's emerging philosophy of hiring community organizer/planners to work with educators, we hoped the group would become self-sustaining and leave the AAC. Despite various efforts to separate, the group never chose to leave and continues today as a semi-autonomous project of AAC. Men join for some period of time, then move on to other projects. Some of the group's activities are fairly routine, while members continue to think up new projects to respond to changes in the local community. Steve Colarusso continues to be the main source of continuity in the project.

3. The two women were Sandy and me. We had hoped to extend the project to

Notes
___

167

include an affinity group of lesbian/bisexual women who would work in the women's bars and social venues. While the men in the project came to accept our participation, even considering us experts on the local gay male community, and while they eagerly passed out dental dams and learned about women's issues in order to talk with women attending functions where the group was doing work, the expansion never succeeded, for reasons that still somewhat elude me. AAC also had a women's project at that time, which was supportive of a safe sex affinity group, but the two projects never meshed. I still believe that the barriers between lesbian/bisexual women's and gay males' sexual issues, and between lesbian/bisexual women's and heterosexual women's sexual issues, were exacerbated by the perception that safe sex education was an emergency that did not include lesbians. I have a more extensive discussion of the problems surrounding lesbians and AIDS in my *Last Served?* (1994).

4. The reading list included Gayle Rubin's "Thinking Sex," John d'Emilio's *Sexual Politics/Sexual Communities,* and my *Sex and Germs: The Politics of* AIDS. The group conveners, which included volunteers Chris LaCharite and Sandy McCloud along with Steve Colarusso and me, who were staff members of AAC, were also influenced by Paulo Freire's work on radical pedagogy.

5. In fact, gay and straight porn now look remarkably similar, not least because many companies produce both using the same actors. Both rely heavily on a narrow range of sexual activities — mainly oral sex and fucking — and close-ups of intercourse interrupted (completed?) by a copious come shot.

6. This description of interpretive schemes was published in an earlier version. Unlike much of the rest of the analysis of these debates, which has also been published in other places but is edited and sometimes completely changed here, I have retained the next section almost exactly as I wrote it in 1989. Although of course my method of tracking these debates is deeply personally invested and hardly ethnographically valid, I keep these sections intact as a document of what I thought participants were saying at the time. I revised this section several times in the months after we debated the video project. I gave the first account of these occurrences as a paper at a hugely attended session at the Fifth International Conference on AIDS in Montreal (we had an overflow hall of thousands, plus closed circuit television — which was blacked out when the actual "porn" video examples were shown). On that occasion, the videos included the first two GMHC videos and a series, produced by Wieland Speck, to be appended to pornography imported into Germany.

7. The following general designations are based on my own casual and unsystematic observations in dozens of ordinary video stores, as well as ones that specialized in "erotica" but were not in zoned sex areas. The stores had roughly the same type of, and often even the same specific, videos. Often, they stocked the entire line — gay, straight, bi (usually lesbian videos come from specialized houses) — from particular produc-

Notes

168

tion companies. I examined both the box covers and a sampling of the videos they contained.

8. As I have argued at length, the U.S. national strategies had devastating consequences internationally in three ways: the initial U.S. framing of the disease as related to homosexuality was adopted elsewhere, even when the demographic configuration of cases was clearly different; the notions of health and disease that underwrote the very definition of AIDS — a deadly malfunction in otherwise healthy persons — made it difficult to distinguish AIDS from other disorders in places with more depressed health profiles and already prevalent wasting diseases; the arrogant privileging of U.S. lives meant that the United States, and to a lesser extent the WHO, was willing to sacrifice local health needs elsewhere in service of scientific research that largely benefited the United States.

Conclusion: From Visibility to Insurrection: A Manifesto

1. The Human Rights Campaign Fund's recent adoption of Gingrich's lesbian half-sister will not only not neutralize him, it will reify the idea of family that has been so devastating to queer politics. Homosexuality becomes an issue over which mutually loving family members can disagree. I am reminded of Frederick Douglass's notorious refusal to debate the issue of slavery in his efforts at abolition. Some things are not debatable, and to treat them as an "issue" is to lay the ground for your own defeat. To *debate* obscures the fact that a policy disagreement is never an "honest disagreement," but a case of moral differences undergirded by real differences in power.

2. Bourdieu (1972) emphasizes the point that the practice is ineffable — if we give an account of our practice we will inevitably misexplain how we do what we do, and worse, how we know what it is we do. This is not really a crisis for those of us who want to stop people from fucking without condoms. They already know how and why they practice in this way, so they must already know how and why they could practice in another way. It may be that the difficulty in practicing differently is that we try to route "change" through cognition. The horrific overemphasis on cognitive processing in the service of producing "safe sex" may have disabled the very disposition, experienced as bodily desires — what Bourdieu calls body hexis to indicate the body knowledges that we wear like skin — that would have had what we have named "safe sex" as their practical, logical expression. It is these dispositions that I am suggesting we try to rediscover, not through more cognitive activities or theoretical theories, but as practical theories, as the complex of possible erotic practices that our bodies *already know.*

3. We need not construct an ethic that valorizes any and all policed sexualities just because we do not yet have a basis for deciding conflicts over sexual rhetorics and the

harms and privileges they claim. I can be relatively clear that Jesse Helms is trying to suppress legitimate sexual vernaculars, even if I am still uncertain how — or
whether — to resolve the conflicts over access to and control over the narrow space of
sexual expression and sexual safety that sometimes collide and sometimes reinforce
each other in the narrow space of "my community." Can we not distinguish between
our common outrage at Helms and the diverse and conflicting outrage at the *GO* ad I
discussed in the introduction? Can we not imagine ways of keeping Helms's hands out
of our business, even while we work toward better ways to critique and learn across
our own divisions and vernaculars?

4. For the most part, anti-essentialist *historical* arguments have relied on Foucault's
History of Sexuality, which, while convincing, leaves several questions unanswered:
for example, how individual bodies take up the notion of essence, and why that idea —
even though we can see its problems — remains personally vital. Bourdieu's concept of
body hexis offers suggestive ways to fill out the descriptive gaps in Foucault's micro-
physics. Parallel with Foucault, Bourdieu argues that body hexis, or the phenom-
enologic sense of self-materiality, always confuses ontology with *location* in the grid
of fields of struggle and in the social space of fractional capital accumulation. The
sense of where you are, of emplacement, which is so evident in cruising, is lost in the
shift into the register of queer codes precisely because they are carried as body hexis,
as dispositions respective to a particular field. But, Bourdieu might offer in defense of
Foucault's general historical argument, we mistake the abstract or virtual social location for an internal quality, or essence: the feeling of "presence" that is actually our
enduring sense of being located in a struggle over values is interiorized (perhaps
because a theoretical discourse is demanded of it) as an element present *in* the body.

Notes

170

Bibliography

Abelove, Henry. 1992. "Some Speculations on the History of 'Sexual Intercourse' during the 'Long Eighteenth Century' in England." *Nationalisms and Sexualities.* Ed. Andrew Parker, Mary Russo, Doris Sommer, and Patricia Yaeger. New York: Routledge.

———. 1993. "From Thoreau to Queer Politics." *Yale Journal of Criticism,* Vol. 6, No. 2.

Abelove, Henry, David Halperin, and Michèle Barale, 1993. *The Lesbian and Gay Studies Reader.* New York: Routledge.

Abrams, Dominic, Charles Abraham, Russell Spears, and Deborah Marks. 1990. "AIDS Invulnerability: Relationships, Sexual Behavior and Attitudes among 16–19 Year Olds." *AIDS: Individual, Cultural and Policy Dimensions.* Ed. Peter Aggleton, Peter Davies, and Graham Hart. Bristol, Penn.: Falmer Press.

Aggleton, Peter, Hilary Homans, Jan Mojsa, Stuart Watson, and Simon Watney. 1989. *AIDS: Scientific and Social Issues, A Resource for Health Educators.* London: Churchill Livingston.

Althusser, Louis. 1977. *Lenin and Philosophy and Other Essays.* London: Verso.

Anderson, Benedict. 1991. *Imagined Communities.* London: Verso.

Athey, Jean L. 1991. "HIV Infection and Homeless Adolescents." *Child Welfare,* Vol. 70, No. 5.

Bandy, P., and P. A. President. 1983. "Recent Literature on Drug Abuse Prevention and Mass Media: Focusing on Youth, Parents, Women and the Elderly." *Journal of Drug Education,* Vol. 13.

Barber, J. G., R. Bradshaw, and C. Walsh. 1989. "Reducing Alcohol Consumption through Television Advertising." *Journal of Consulting and Clinical Psychology,* Vol. 57.

Battjes, Robert J., and Roy W. Pickens. 1988. "Needle Sharing among Intravenous Drug Abusers." National Institutes of Drug Abuse Monograph 80.

Baudrillard, Jean. 1987. *The Ecstasy of Communication.* New York: Semiotext(e).

Bhahba, Homi. 1983. "The Other Question: The Stereotype and Colonial Discourse." *Screen,* Vol. 26, No. 6.

Black, G. S. 1988. *The Attitudinal Basis for Drug Use — 1987 and Changing Attitudes toward Drug Use — 1988.* Reports from the Media-Advertising Partnership for a Drug-Free America, Inc. Rochester, N.Y.: Gordon S. Black.

Boston AIDS Consortium. 1991. *Community Voices: A Compilation of Public Testimony by People with HIV Disease and Care Providers.* Boston: Boston AIDS Consortium.

Bourdieu, Pierre. 1972. *Outline for a Theory of Practice.* Cambridge: Cambridge University Press.

Boyer, Cherrie B., and Susan M. Kegeles. 1991. "AIDS Risk and Prevention among Adolescents." *Social Science Medicine,* Vol. 33, No. 1.

Bromley, David G., and Charles F. Longino Jr., eds. 1972. *White Racism and Black Americans.* Cambridge, Mass.: Schenkman Publishing.

Brownworth, Victoria A. 1992. "Teen Sex: America's Worst-Kept Secret." *The Advocate,* Issue 599, March.

Burroughs-Wellcome. 1989. *HIV Counselling.* Research Triangle Park, N.C.

Butler, J. 1990. *Gender Trouble: Feminism and the Subversion of Identity.* New York: Routledge.

Caplan, Pat, ed. 1987. *The Cultural Construction of Sexuality.* London: Tavistock.

Coates, Thomas J. 1990. "Strategies for Modifying Sexual Behavior for Primary and Secondary Prevention of HIV Disease." *Journal of Consulting and Clinical Psychology,* Vol. 58, No. 1.

Commonwealth of Massachusetts Department of Education (CMDE). 1990. "1990 Massachusetts Youth Risk Behavior Survey Results."

Commonwealth of Massachusetts Department of Public Health (CMDPH). 1990. "Adolescents at Risk: Sexually Transmitted Diseases."

D'Emilio, John. 1983. *Sexual Politics/Sexual Communities.* Chicago: University of Chicago Press.

Department of Health and Hospitals (DHH). 1992. "HIV and Boston's Adolescents: A Report on the Impending Public Health Crisis."

Des Jarlais, Don C., Samuel R. Friedman, and Cathy Casriel. 1990. "Target Groups for Preventing AIDS among Intravenous Drug Users: 2. The 'Hard' Data Studies." *Journal of Consulting and Clinical Psychology,* Vol. 58, No. 1.

Dollimore, Jonathan. 1992. *Sexual Dissidence: Augustine to Wilde, Freud to Foucault.* New York: Oxford University Press.

Bibliography

Duggan, Lisa. 1992. "Making It Perfectly Queer." *Socialist Review,* Spring.

Duggan, Lisa, and Nan Hunter. 1995. *Sex Wars: Sexual Dissent and Political Culture.* New York: Routledge.

Eckholm, Erik. 1990. "Cut down as They Grow up: AIDS Stalks Gay Teen-Agers." *New York Times,* December 13.

Elkind, David. 1990. "What Teens Know about AIDS." *Parents,* March.

Fettner, Ann Guidici, and William A. Check. 1984. *The Truth about AIDS: Evolution of an Epidemic.* New York: Holt, Rinehart, and Winston.

Foucault, Michel. 1972. *Archeology of Knowledge.* New York: Pantheon.

———. 1980. *The History of Sexuality, Introduction.* New York: Vintage.

Frank, Judith. 1995. " 'To Sir With Love': National Pedagogy in the Clinton Era." *Higher Education Under Fire: Politics, Economics, and the Crisis of the Humanities.* Ed. Michael Bérubé and Cary Nelson. New York: Routledge.

Freire, Paulo. 1973. *Education for Critical Consciousness.* New York: Seabury Press.

Freud, Anna. 1958. "Adolescence." *Psychoanalytic Study of the Child.* New York: International Universities Press.

Freud, Sigmund. 1963. *Three Essays on the Theory of Sexuality.* New York: Basic Books.

———. "The Taboo of Virginity." 1974. *Sexuality and the Psychology of Love.* New York: Collier.

Fry, V., A. Alexander, and D. Fry. 1990. "Textual Status, the Stigmatized Self, and Media Consumption." *Communication Yearbook,* Issue 13. Ed. James Anderson. Newbury Park, Calif.: Sage.

Glendhill, C. 1988. "Pleasurable Negotiations." *Female Spectators: Looking at Film and Television.* Ed. E. Deidre Pribram. London: Verso.

Good Housekeeping. 1990. "Teenagers and AIDS," May.

Gross, Jane. 1987. "AIDS Threat Brings New Turmoil for Gay Teen-Agers." *New York Times,* October 21.

Hamburg, David A., and Ruby Takanishi. 1989. "Preparing for Life: The Critical Transition of Adolescence." *American Psychologist,* Vol. 44, No. 5.

Hammersly, Martyn, and Paul Atkinson. 1983. *Ethnography Principles in Practice.* London: Routledge.

Hebdige, Dick. 1979. *Subculture: The Meaning of Style.* New York: Routledge, Chapman and Hall.

Hersch, Patricia. 1988. "Coming of Age on City Streets." *Psychology Today,* January.

Hingson, Robert, et al. 1990. "Beliefs about AIDS, Use of Alcohol and Drugs, and Unprotected Sex among Massachusetts Adolescents." *American Journal of Public Health,* Vol. 80, No. 3.

Kolata, Gina. 1990. "Teenagers and AIDS." *Seventeen,* May.

Bibliography

Jackson, Anthony W. and David W. Hornbeck. 1989. "Educating Young Adolescents: Why We Must Restructure Middle Grade Schools." *American Psychologist,* Vol. 44, No. 5 (May).

McRobbie, Angela. 1991. *Feminism and Youth Culture: From "Jackie" to "Just Seventeen."* London: Macmillan.

Mead, Margaret. 1935. *Sex and Temperament in Three Primitive Societies.* New York: William Morrow.

Memon, Amina. 1991. "Perceptions of Vulnerability: The Role of Attributions and Social Context." *AIDS: Responses, Interventions and Care.* Ed. Peter Aggleton, Graham Hart, and Peter Davis. Bristol, Penn.: Falmer Press.

Miller, Brent C., Roger B. Christensen, and Terrance D. Olson. 1987. "Adolescent Self-Esteem in Relation to Sexual Attitudes and Behavior." *Youth and Society,* Vol. 19, No. 1 (September).

Modeleski, Tania. 1984. *Loving with a Vengeance: Mass-produced Fantasies for Women.* Methuen: London.

Mulvey, Laura. 1989. *Visual and Other Pleasures.* Bloomington: Indiana University Press.

National Institute on Drug Abuse. 1990. "The Collection and Interpretation of Data from Hidden Populations." National Institutes of Drug Abuse Monograph 98.

Neale, Steve. 1983. "Masculinity as Spectacle." *Screen,* Vol. 24, No. 6.

Nelson, Jenny. 1989. "Eyes out of Your Head: On Televisual Experience." *Critical Studies in Mass Communication,* Vol. 6, No. 4 (December).

Newsweek. 1985. "Campus Sex: New Fears," October 28.

———. 1990. "The Future of Gay America," March 12.

Nordheimer, Jon. 1987. "AIDS Specter for Women: The Bisexual Man." *New York Times,* April 8.

Pajaczkowska, Claire. 1981. "The Heterosexual Presumption: A Contribution to the Debate on Pornography." *Screen,* Vol. 22, No. 1.

Patton, Cindy. 1985a. "Heterosexual AIDS Panic: A Queer Paradigm." *Gay Community News,* February 9.

———. 1985b. *Sex and Germs: The Politics of AIDS.* Boston: South End Press.

———. 1988. "The Cum Shot—Three Takes on Lesbian and Gay Sexuality." *OUT/LOOK,* Fall.

———. 1990. *Inventing AIDS.* New York: Routledge.

———. 1992a. "From Nation to Family: Containing African AIDS." *Nationalisms and Sexualities.* Ed. Andrew Parker, Mary Russo, Doris Sommer, and Patricia Yaeger. New York: Routledge.

———. 1992b. " 'With Champagne and Roses': Women at Risk from/in AIDS Discourse." *Women and AIDS*. Ed. Corrine Squire. Sage Women and Psychology Series. London: Sage.

——. 1992c. "Fear of AIDS: The Erotics of Innocence and Ingenuity." *American Imago,* winter 1993.

——. 1994. *Last Served? Gendering the HIV Pandemic*. London: Falmer.

——. 1995a. "Forward to the New Edition." *Lavender Culture*. Ed. Karla Jay and Allen Young. New York: New York University Press.

——. 1995b. "Refiguring Social Space." *Social Postmodernism*. Ed. Linda Nicholson and Steven Seidman. Cambridge: Cambridge University Press.

——. 1995c. "Between Innocence and Safety: Representations of Young People's Need to Know about 'Safe Sex.' " *Deviant Bodies*. Ed. Jacqueline Urla and Jennifer Terry. Bloomington: Indiana University Press.

Powers, Sally I., Stuart T. Hauser, and Linda A. Kilner. 1989. "Adolescent Mental Health." *American Psychologist,* Vol. 44, No. 2.

Price, Stephen. 1988. "The Pornographic Image and the Practice of Film Theory." *Cinema Journal,* Vol. 27, No. 2 (winter).

Radway, Janice. 1983. "Women Read the Romance: The Interpretation of Text and Context." *Feminist Studies,* Vol. 9, No. 1 (spring).

Ramos, Reyes. 1990. "Chicano Intravenous Drug Users." National Institutes of Drug Abuse Monograph 98.

Roberts, Wallace, ed. 1971. *The Little Red Schoolbook*. New York: Pocket Books.

Rosenbaum, Marsha, and Sheigla Murphy. 1990. "Women and Addiction: Process, Treatment, and Outcome." National Institutes of Drug Abuse Monograph 98.

Rubin, A. M. 1984. "Ritualized and Instrumental Television Viewing." *Journal of Communication,* Vol. 34, No. 3.

Rubin, Gayle. 1984. "Thinking Sex." *Pleasure and Danger*. Ed. Carole Vance. Boston: Routledge and Kegan Paul.

Russo, Vito. 1981. *The Celluloid Closet*. New York: Harper and Row.

Said, Edward. 1978. *Orientalism*. New York: Pantheon.

Schilling, Robert F., and Alfred L. McAlister. 1990. "Preventing Drug Use in Adolescents through Media Interventions." *Journal of Consulting and Clinical Psychology,* Vol. 58, No. 4.

Sedgwick, E. 1990. *The Epistemology of the Closet*. Berkeley: University of California Press.

Strauss, Anselm, and Juliet Corbin. 1990. *Basics of Qualitative Research*. Newbury Park, Calif.: Sage.

Surgeon General. 1988. "Understanding AIDS." Washington: Government Printing Office.

Swanson, Nancy, Kathryn Lasch, Cindy Patton, and Fuat Yalin. 1991. "HIV Counseling and Testing Evaluation Study: Ethnographic Component." Unpublished report. Atlanta: Centers for Disease Control.

Time. 1985a. "The AIDS Issue Hits the Schools," September 9.

——. 1985b. "The New Untouchables," September 23.

——. 1986. "Lessening Fears," February 17.

Turner, Victor. 1967. *The Forest of Symbols.* Ithaca: Cornell University Press.

Van Gelder, Lindsy, and Pam Brandt. 1986. "AIDS on Campus." *Rolling Stone,* Issue 483, September 25.

Weeks, Jeffrey. 1986. *Sexuality.* London: Tavistock.

Welling, Kay. 1989. "Preliminary Report on a Pilot Study." Social Aspects of AIDS Conference, South Bank Polytechnique Institute, London.

Wilton, Tamsin, and Peter Aggleton. 1991. "Condoms, Coercion and Control: Hetero-sexuality and the Limits to HIV/AIDS Education." *AIDS: Responses, Interventions and Care.* Ed. Peter Aggleton, Graham Hart, and Peter Davis. Bristol, Penn.: Falmer Press.

Yarrow, Andrew L. 1989. "Putting the AIDS Message Where the Trouble Is." *New York Times,* September 13.

Bibliography

Index

New technology, 17
1970s, 10, 13, 19, 63, 109–10

Parker, Al, 122–24
Pornography, 5, 6, 78, 111, 117, 127–38,
    146; home video, 129–33, 144–45
Power, 9, 18, 52

Queer Nation, 11, 19, 139

Radical feminism, 4, 5
Relapse, 109
Right-wing, 34, 118, 141, 144–45, 154
Risk: perceptions of, 36, 65

"Safe Company," 120–27
Safe sex: and communication, 105–6, 110,
    143, 147; as emancipation, 108–12; and
    heterosexuality, 19, 28, 73; "Hot,
    Horny, and Healthy" workshop, 105–7,
    112; interpretations of, 3, 4, 6, 7, 17, 23,
    28, 29, 34, 54, 81, 100–101, 107, 117,
    119, 124–27; as a norm, 108–10, 120;
    partner selection strategy, 28–30, 80,
    83, 101, 104; pornographic examples
    of, 133–37

Savitz, Edward ("Uncle Eddie"), 23, 63–
    83
Sexual compulsivity, 104–5
Sexual explicitness: problems with, 115–
    17, 145–46
Sexuality and space, 143, 145, 147–53
Sexual perversion: concepts of, 67–70
Sexual representation, 6, 12–17, 124–
    27
Sexual vernacular, 98, 142–45, 146–47,
    153
Sexual violence, 5
Stop AIDS Project, 107–8
Surgeon General's report, 11, 145

White, Ryan, 8, 25, 41, 71

Youth, 34, 37–38; adult's attitudes toward,
    38, 51, 55, 62, 74; of color, 37, 42–43,
    50, 57–62; and drug injection, 40; gay,
    42–43, 53–57, 61–62; HIV seropreva-
    lence among, 35–36, 39–40; knowl-
    edge about HIV, 39–40; perceptions of
    risk for HIV, 39–40; and sexuality, 36–
    38; storm and stress theory of, 37, 43–
    46, 75; as subculture, 37, 49–53

About the Author

Cindy Patton is Assistant Professor in the Department of English at Temple University. She is the author of *Last Served?: Gendering the HIV Pandemic, Inventing AIDS, Making It: A Woman's Guide to Sex in the Age of AIDS,* and *Sex and Germs: The Politics of AIDS.*

Library of Congress Cataloging-in-Publication Data

Patton, Cindy.

Fatal advice / by Cindy Patton.

p. cm. — (Series Q)

Includes bibliographical references and index.

ISBN 0-8223-1750-8 (cl : alk. paper). — ISBN 0-8223-1747-8 (pa : alk. paper)

1. Sex instruction — United States. 2. Hygiene, Sexual — Study and

teaching — United States. 3. Safe sex in AIDS prevention — Study and

teaching — United States. I. Title. II. Series.

HQ57.5.A3P37 1996

613.9'07 — dc20   95-44292

CIP